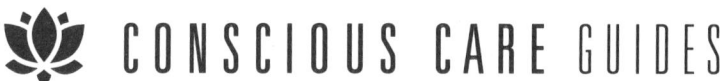

# Cognitive Behavioral Therapy

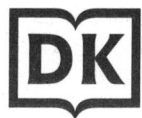

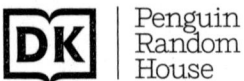

**Publisher:** Mike Sanders
**Senior Acquisitions Editor:** Jan Lynn
**Art Director:** William Thomas
**Copy Editor:** Rick Kughen
**Cover/Book Designer:** William Thomas
**Layout:** Ayanna Lacey
**Proofreader:** Monica Stone
**Indexer:** Celia McCoy

*This book is dedicated to my dear husband, Keith, for his patience and support in all my pursuits. B and L.*
*—Jayme Albin*

*Dedicated to my daughter, Evelyn.*
*You bring sunshine into my life every day.*
*I love you.*
*—Eileen Bailey*

First American Edition, 2021
Published in the United States by DK Publishing
6081 E. 82nd Street, Indianapolis, IN 46250

Copyright © 2021 Dorling Kindersley Limited
DK, a Division of Penguin Random House LLC
21 22 23 10 9 8 7 6 5 4 3 2 1
001-322009-MAR2021

All rights reserved.
Without limiting the rights under the copyright reserved above, no part of this publication may be reproduced, stored in or introduced into a retrieval system, or transmitted, in any form, or by any means (electronic, mechanical, photocopying, recording, or otherwise), without the prior written permission of the copyright owner.
Published in Great Britain by Dorling Kindersley Limited

Library of Congress Catalog Number: 2020941357
ISBN 978-1-61564-985-3

DK books are available at special discounts when purchased in bulk for sales promotions, premiums, fund-raising, or educational use. For details, contact: DK Publishing Special Markets,
1450 Broadway, Suite 801, New York, NY 10018
SpecialSales@dk.com

Printed and bound in the United States of America

**For the curious**
**www.dk.com**

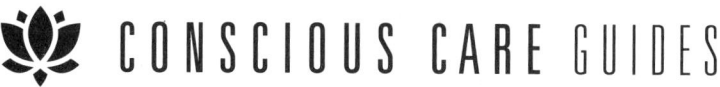

# Cognitive Behavioral Therapy

Dr. Jayme Albin and Eileen Bailey

Reprinted and updated from *Idiot's Guides®: Cognitive Behavioral Therapy*

# Contents

## Part 1: The Basics of Cognitive Behavioral Therapy ..................................................1

### Chapter 1: Understanding CBT ......................................................................... 3
What Is CBT? ........................................................................................................ 3
What Are Automatic Thoughts? ........................................................................... 3
What Are Core Beliefs? ........................................................................................ 4
Your Turn: What Kind of Thinker Are You? ........................................................ 5
Seven Myths You Might Believe About CBT ...................................................... 5
The Theory Behind CBT ....................................................................................... 7
Your Turn: Learning Your ABCs .......................................................................... 8
Understanding Themes ......................................................................................... 9
Benefits of CBT ................................................................................................... 10
Disadvantages of CBT ........................................................................................ 10
Comparing CBT to Other Forms of Therapy .................................................... 11
Your Turn: Is CBT Right for Me? ....................................................................... 12

### Chapter 2: Interpreting Your Thoughts and Feelings ................................... 15
Thoughts, Feelings, and Behaviors .................................................................... 15
Your Turn: New Beliefs ...................................................................................... 18
Separating Thoughts from Emotions ................................................................. 18
Problematic Thought Processes ........................................................................ 20
Your Turn: Notice Your Thoughts ...................................................................... 25

### Chapter 3: Automatic Thoughts, Assumptions, and Core Beliefs ............... 27
Your First Reaction ............................................................................................. 27
Your Turn: Listening to Self-Talk ....................................................................... 28
Negative Automatic Thoughts ........................................................................... 28
Changing Negative Self-Talk ............................................................................. 29
Your Turn: Questions to Ask Yourself ............................................................... 31
Making Assumptions .......................................................................................... 31
Your Turn: Turning Assumptions Around ......................................................... 32
Tips for Eliminating Assumptions ...................................................................... 33
Your Turn: Uncovering Your Assumptions ....................................................... 34
Identify Your Core Beliefs .................................................................................. 35
Your Turn: Rating Core Beliefs .......................................................................... 36
Develop New Core Beliefs ................................................................................. 37

## Chapter 4: Understanding and Measuring Your Emotions .......... 39
Naming Your Emotions .......... 39
Helpful vs. Unhelpful Emotions .......... 40
Your Turn: Discover Underlying Attitudes .......... 44
Mixed Emotions .......... 45
Managing Feelings about Feelings .......... 46
Your Turn: Create an Emotion Contract .......... 46
The Emotional Process .......... 47
Cognitive Reactions .......... 47
Physical Reactions .......... 48
Behavioral Reactions .......... 49
Learned Emotions .......... 49

# Part 2: CBT Techniques .......... 53

## Chapter 5: Setting Goals for Getting Better .......... 55
Setting Goals .......... 55
Your Turn: Ladder Rungs .......... 57
Define Your Motivation .......... 58
Making Sure the Goal Is Yours .......... 60
Your Turn: Create a Cost-Benefit Analysis .......... 60
Your Turn: Create Coping Flash Cards .......... 61
Maintaining Your Progress .......... 61
Tips for Setting Goals .......... 62

## Chapter 6: Visualization and Imagery .......... 63
Using Visualization .......... 63
Facing Emotional Images .......... 64
Reacting to Spontaneous Imagery .......... 65
Your Turn: Create Your Imagery .......... 68
Create Coping Skills .......... 68
Your Turn: Keynote-Behavior Visualizations .......... 69

## Chapter 7: Relaxation Techniques and Strategies .......... 71
The Importance of Breathing .......... 71
Your Turn: Breathing Techniques .......... 72
Your Turn: Simple Meditation .......... 75
Your Turn: Kirtan Kriya Meditation .......... 76
Relaxing Your Muscles .......... 76

Your Turn: Progressive Muscle Relaxation ......................................................................... 77
Other Ways to Relax .............................................................................................................. 78
Your Turn: Create a Wish List ................................................................................................ 79
Your Turn: Activity Journal ..................................................................................................... 81

## Chapter 8: Mindfulness ........................................................................................ 83
What Is Mindfulness? ............................................................................................................. 83
Your Turn: Mindfulness Breathing ......................................................................................... 84
A Thought Is Just a Thought .................................................................................................. 84
The Role of Mindfulness in CBT ............................................................................................ 85
Controlling Urges .................................................................................................................... 85
Your Turn: The Raisin Experience ......................................................................................... 86
Being Present in the Moment ................................................................................................. 86
Tips for Living in the Present Moment ................................................................................... 87
Watch Your Thoughts Sail By ................................................................................................. 88
Your Turn: Observing Thoughts ............................................................................................. 88
Accepting Upsetting Thoughts and Moods ........................................................................... 88
Incorporating Mindfulness in Everyday Life ........................................................................... 89
Your Turn: Diary of Mindfulness Exercises ............................................................................ 90

## Chapter 9: Your Inner Narration ........................................................................... 91
Self-Talk ................................................................................................................................... 91
Your Turn: Recording Your Inner Dialogue ............................................................................ 92
Types of Negative Narrations ................................................................................................. 93
Checklist for More Positive Inner Narration ........................................................................... 95
Your Turn: Which Category? .................................................................................................. 95
Affirmations ............................................................................................................................. 96
Combating the Idea of Lying to Yourself ............................................................................... 96
Tips for Creating Affirmations ................................................................................................ 98

## Chapter 10: Testing Your New Beliefs .................................................................. 99
Reality Testing ......................................................................................................................... 99
Comparing Behaviors ........................................................................................................... 101
Feedback ............................................................................................................................... 103
Your Turn: Testing Your Predictions .................................................................................... 106

## Part 3: CBT for Personal Growth ............................................................. 107

### Chapter 11: Increasing Your Self-Esteem ................................................ 109
What Do We Mean by Self-Esteem? ........................................................... 109
Self-Acceptance ......................................................................................... 109
Obstacles to Self-Acceptance ................................................................... 110
Your Turn: Self-Assessment ...................................................................... 112
Steps to Improving Self-Esteem ................................................................ 112
Your Turn: Create Mini Action Plans ......................................................... 114

### Chapter 12: Overcoming Perfectionism ................................................. 117
Defining Perfectionism .............................................................................. 117
Your Turn: Are You a Perfectionist? .......................................................... 118
Perfectionist Thought Patterns ................................................................. 119
Adding Flexibility to Your Life ................................................................... 120
Your Turn: Shades of Gray ........................................................................ 123
Cost-Benefit Analysis ................................................................................ 123
Procrastination and Perfectionism ........................................................... 124
Your Turn: Taking One Step at a Time ...................................................... 125

### Chapter 13: Improving Your Relationships ............................................ 127
Who Is to Blame? ....................................................................................... 127
Communication Skills ............................................................................... 131

### Chapter 14: Building Assertiveness ....................................................... 135
Defining Assertiveness .............................................................................. 135
Steps for Assertiveness ............................................................................. 136
Types of Assertiveness .............................................................................. 139
Acting Assertively ...................................................................................... 142
Accepting Criticism ................................................................................... 143
Misconceptions About Assertiveness ...................................................... 144

### Chapter 15: Managing Everyday Stress ................................................. 145
What Is Stress? .......................................................................................... 145
Identify Your Stressors .............................................................................. 146
Problems vs. Problematic Thinking .......................................................... 147
Your Turn: Problem Solving ...................................................................... 148
Stress Reduction Strategies ..................................................................... 149
Your Turn: Create a Stress Worksheet ..................................................... 150
Exercise Your Stress Away ........................................................................ 151

## Part 4: CBT for Specific Conditions and Situations .................................................. 153

### Chapter 16: Overcoming Depression .......................................................... 155
Sadness vs. Depression ............................................................................. 155
The Role of CBT in Treating Depression ................................................... 156
The "Do Nothing" Syndrome ..................................................................... 158
Avoidance .................................................................................................. 159
Ruminations .............................................................................................. 160
Your Turn: Reduce Your Ruminations ....................................................... 161
Take Care of Yourself ................................................................................ 163

### Chapter 17: Dealing with Anxiety Disorders .............................................. 167
Types of Anxiety Disorders ........................................................................ 167
The Role of CBT in Treating Anxiety Disorders ........................................ 168
Facing Fears .............................................................................................. 169
Your Turn: Expose Yourself ....................................................................... 171
Turn Worry into Problem Solving .............................................................. 171
Accepting Uncertainty ............................................................................... 172
Your Turn: Create a Worry Script .............................................................. 173
Your Turn: Managing Big Problems ........................................................... 173
Behavior Assignments ............................................................................... 174

### Chapter 18: Controlling Anger .................................................................. 177
What Is Anger? .......................................................................................... 177
Understanding Your Anger ........................................................................ 177
Healthy vs. Unhealthy Anger .................................................................... 181
Your Turn: How Angry Are You? ............................................................... 183
Common Hot Buttons ................................................................................ 183
Reframe Your Emotion .............................................................................. 185
Accept Fallibility in Yourself and Others ................................................... 185
Your Turn: Judge Yourself First ................................................................ 186
Increase Your Frustration Tolerance ......................................................... 186
Your Turn: Raise Your Frustration Tolerance ........................................... 187

### Chapter 19: Managing OCD ....................................................................... 189
Understanding Obsessive-Compulsive Disorder ....................................... 189
Your Turn: Identify Your Triggers ............................................................. 191
Thoughts Are Just Thoughts ..................................................................... 192
Your Turn: Thought Exposure ................................................................... 192
Overcoming Magical Thinking ................................................................... 192
Response Prevention ................................................................................. 193

Behavioral Experiments ................................................................................................. 193
Exposure Therapy .......................................................................................................... 194
Tips for Reducing Rituals .............................................................................................. 195
Build on Successes ........................................................................................................ 196

## Chapter 20: Developing a Positive Body Image ............................................ 199
What Is Body Image? .................................................................................................... 199
Healthy vs. Unhealthy Body Image .............................................................................. 199
Your Turn: Do You Have a Body Image Problem? ..................................................... 200
Problematic Thinking Processes .................................................................................. 201
Your Turn: Changing the Image ................................................................................... 202
How Body Image Affects Your Life ............................................................................. 202
Your Turn: The Real Impact ......................................................................................... 203
Standing in Your Way ................................................................................................... 204
See Yourself as a Whole Person .................................................................................. 205
A Word About Eating Disorders .................................................................................. 206

## Chapter 21: CBT for Grief .................................................................................. 209
What Is Grief? ................................................................................................................ 209
Your Turn: How Does Grief Affect You? .................................................................... 210
Allow Yourself to Grieve .............................................................................................. 211
The Psychology of Grief ............................................................................................... 211
Your Turn: Mixed Emotions ......................................................................................... 212
Death Can Challenge Your Beliefs About the World ................................................. 212
There Is Loss of More than Just a Person ................................................................... 213
How CBT Helps ............................................................................................................. 214
Your Turn: Listen to Your Story .................................................................................. 217
Getting Through Waves of Grief ................................................................................. 217
Your Turn: Writing a Letter .......................................................................................... 218
Uncomplicated vs. Complicated Grief ........................................................................ 218

## Chapter 22: Physical Illness ............................................................................... 221
How Does CBT Help with Physical Illness? ............................................................... 221
Living with Diabetes ..................................................................................................... 222
Your Turn: Problem Solving to Eliminate Barriers to Treatment Compliance ........ 223
Managing Chronic Pain ................................................................................................. 224
Heart Disease ................................................................................................................. 226
Your Turn: Dissecting Procrastination ........................................................................ 227
Menopause ..................................................................................................................... 228
Your Turn: Practice Mindfulness ................................................................................. 229

Insomnia..................................................................................................................229
Gastrointestinal Disorders.................................................................................231
Your Turn: Decatastrophizing............................................................................232

# Part 5: Moving Forward .................................................................233

## Chapter 23: Knocking Down Obstacles to Progress ................................. 235
Uncovering More Problems and Feeling Overwhelmed.......................................235
Common Reasons CBT Doesn't Work ...............................................................236
Getting in Your Way..........................................................................................239
Your Turn: Find Your Motivation .......................................................................241
Monitor Your Progress ......................................................................................241
Tips to Make CBT Work for You .......................................................................242

## Chapter 24: Maintaining Gains ................................................................ 243
Prepare for Triggers: CBT as Part of a Healthy Lifestyle .....................................244

## Chapter 25: Preparing to Backslide.......................................................... 247
The Difference Between a Lapse and a Relapse .................................................247
Your Turn: Preparing for a Setback ...................................................................248
Warning Signs and Triggers ..............................................................................249
Your Turn: Create a Relapse Prevention Plan ....................................................250
Tips for Integrating CBT into Daily Life .............................................................251

## Chapter 26: Internet-Delivered CBT (iCBT)............................................. 253
How Does Internet-Delivered CBT Work?..........................................................253
The Pros and Cons ...........................................................................................255
Where to Find iCBT Programs ..........................................................................256
Five E-Therapy Websites...................................................................................258
Five Online CBT Programs ...............................................................................259
Five Helpful Apps .............................................................................................260

## Chapter 27: Working with a Therapist..................................................... 263
Should You Seek Professional Help?..................................................................263
Conventional Therapy vs. CBT .........................................................................264
Finding a Therapist ..........................................................................................266
Be Prepared to Participate ................................................................................269
A Typical Therapy Session ................................................................................270

Appendix A: Glossary .................................................................................... 273

Appendix B: Resources for Finding a CBT Therapist ....................................281

Appendix C: Forms ........................................................................................ 285

Appendix D: References ............................................................................... 307

Index ...............................................................................................................315

# Introduction

Cognitive-behavioral therapy (CBT) is different from traditional "talk" therapy. You might think of it as working to resolve issues in your past to move forward. CBT, on the other hand, focuses on present-day thought processes, although you do consider the past during the process. It requires your active participation; completing homework assignments allows you to practice skills and techniques in your daily life. When you work with a therapist, you collaboratively work to set goals and prioritize issues.

CBT is effective in treating a range of issues. The methods described in this book help you look at your thoughts, not just as thoughts but also as precursors to emotions and behaviors. Once you understand your thought process, you can change it and view situations and your life differently. CBT shows you how to think in a more positive, healthy, and helpful way.

While CBT is frequently used in treatment for depression and anxiety, you don't have to be "mentally ill" or have a disorder to benefit from it. The strategies used can improve your life in many ways. They can increase self-esteem, overcome anger issues, and improve relationships. When you practice CBT, you change your inner dialogue and get rid of old, outdated, and damaging views of yourself. You let go of perfectionist ideals and better deal with the uncertainty of life. CBT teaches you how to be assertive and manage the inevitable stress in your life.

This book provides self-help exercises to get you on the road to feeling better. However, if you choose to work with a therapist, you can still benefit from this book. Together, you and your therapist go through sections that address your specific concerns, and you can use the exercises as homework assignments.

CBT is a skill-based therapy. You learn techniques for analyzing your thinking patterns, creating new beliefs, and changing your feelings and emotions by identifying the thoughts behind them. You discover how mindfulness, visualization, and relaxation fit into your overall feelings of well-being. As with all new skills, CBT takes practice and commitment. But once you learn these skills, they are transferable to different situations, and you gain a healthier perspective of yourself, your life, and the world around you.

## How This Book Is Organized

This book is a self-help book. It gives explanations of CBT concepts and provides exercises to help you put those concepts into action. We understand you are not a medical professional and don't want to read a book full of medical jargon. For this reason, we tried to keep the focus of this book free of too much CBT terminology. We included a glossary in the back of the book, should you need additional information.

Some of the exercises call for you to complete a form. We include many of these in Appendix C. Any exercise with a corresponding form has a notation. It might be helpful to make copies of those that you use more than once.

**Part 1, Understanding CBT,** covers the basics of CBT. It explains the theory behind CBT and fundamental concepts you need to know to interpret thoughts and feelings. It discusses the most common problematic thinking patterns and teaches you how to identify your thinking processes. We explain the difference between helpful and unhelpful emotions and how your thoughts relate to these emotions. Finally, we help you set goals for getting better.

**Part 2, CBT Techniques,** covers the basic skills you will use throughout this book. You learn how to change your thoughts by changing the images in your mind. Making changes to your thinking can be scary, so we teach you different relaxation and meditation techniques to incorporate in your life. We explain another helpful approach, mindfulness, and give you exercises to help you be present in the moment. You learn how to talk to yourself positively. Finally, you learn techniques for testing the strong beliefs you hold about yourself.

**Part 3, CBT for Personal Growth,** provides information and exercises for using CBT in your everyday life. There are exercises to build self-acceptance and improve your self-image. We discuss how perfectionism often leads to disappointment in life and give you specific ways to create a more balanced view of yourself and your behavior. We focus on helping you improve your relationship by changing how you think and communicate with your significant other. You learn how to be assertive and deal with the daily stress of life.

**Part 4, CBT for Specific Conditions and Situations,** focuses on problems that can interfere with your ability to enjoy life. You complete thought analysis to identify patterns leading to depression and change your thoughts to feel better. CBT is also effective in treating anxiety, and we give you a step-by-step approach to facing your fears and calming your worries. You learn techniques to tame your temper, better manage obsessive-compulsive disorder, and teach you how to see thoughts as merely thoughts, not premonitions of danger. Finally, we help you change how you feel about your body, giving you exercises to improve your body image. We talk about how CBT improves physical illnesses, such as diabetes, heart disease, menopause, and chronic pain, by changing how you interact with health issues.

**Part 5, Moving Forward,** discusses strategies for making CBT work, even after you completed the book. It examines common reasons CBT doesn't work and provides suggestions for overcoming them. We guide you in setting up a self-therapy session to maintain your new skills. And we help you locate online resources, including internet-delivered CBT programs that complement the concepts in this book. Finally, we discuss finding and working with a therapist, and what to expect during a typical CBT therapy session.

## Acknowledgments

**From Dr. Jayme Albin:** I would like to acknowledge Eileen Bailey, my coauthor, for all her hard work. I would also like to thank my clients from over the years, all of whom have helped me grow personally and professionally.

**From Eileen Bailey:** First, I want to thank Evelyn for providing me with a younger perspective. Many thanks to my coauthor, Jayme, who shared her wealth of knowledge and expertise in cognitive behavioral therapy. I want to thank Steve Brodsky for editing the manuscript and providing insight. And much gratitude to Brandon Buechley, Jan Lynn, and Rick Kughen, the editors who helped bring this book from concept to reality and made it the best it could be. And as always, thanks to my agent Marilyn for thinking of me for this project.

## Trademarks

All terms mentioned in this book that are known to be or are suspected of being trademarks or service marks have been appropriately capitalized. Alpha Books and Penguin Random House LLC cannot attest to the accuracy of this information. Use of a term in this book should not be regarded as affecting the validity of any trademark or service mark.

## Disclaimer

This book is meant as a self-help tool. It provides information and exercises to help you make improvements in your life. We discuss a number of medical conditions. This book is not meant to replace medical care.

PART 1

# The Basics of Cognitive Behavioral Therapy

Cognitive-behavioral therapy (CBT) denotes that your thoughts are responsible for your emotions and behaviors. When you pay attention to your thoughts and consciously modify them to reflect a more positive and balanced way of looking at the world, you change your behaviors and feelings as well. This type of therapy began as a treatment for depression. Today, many people use it to improve mental and physical health issues and as a self-improvement tool.

This part explores the theory behind CBT. We discuss the benefits of this type of therapy and help you decide if CBT is right for you. We help you understand how your thoughts, feelings, and behaviors are related; list common thinking errors; and give you questions to ask yourself to find a more balanced and positive perspective.

# CHAPTER 1
# Understanding CBT

You might be wondering what cognitive behavioral therapy is and whether it could help you. This chapter answers those questions by explaining the basic premise behind CBT and examining the advantages and disadvantages of this type of treatment. Finally, we help you decide if this is the right therapy for you.

## What Is CBT?

Cognitive behavioral therapy (CBT) is a type of psychotherapy that focuses on understanding how your thoughts, feelings, and behaviors are related. The process of CBT emphasizes that you can change how you feel and behave by changing how you think. You might believe the external events of your life shape how you feel and act, but that isn't true. It is your thoughts and your interpretation of events that drive your behaviors and feelings.

To best understand CBT, there are two terms you need to know: automatic thoughts and core beliefs.

## What Are Automatic Thoughts?

Automatic thoughts are thoughts that pop into your mind without a conscious effort. While they can be true, they are frequently negative, although they seem plausible. They are often attached to intense or negative feelings. For example, when starting a new job, you might think, "This is going to be hard; I won't ever learn the job," or "Everyone here is going to think I am stupid if I ask questions." You might not even realize you are having these thoughts. We discuss automatic thoughts in more detail in Chapter 3, but for now, you should have a basic understanding of what they are.

# What Are Core Beliefs?

Core beliefs develop over time, usually beginning in childhood but can develop at any time based on significant life events. You maintain these firmly held, rigid beliefs about yourself by looking for evidence to support them and ignoring evidence that challenges them. Examples of core beliefs include "I am stupid," or "I am unlikeable." When interacting with other people, you might notice only negative feedback that reinforces these beliefs and ignore any compliments or successes that show these beliefs are not correct. Chapter 3 explains core beliefs in more detail.

Let's look at two scenarios. As you read them, think about how they are different. Notice that when thoughts change, behaviors and feelings do as well.

**Scenario 1:** Imagine you have been looking for a job for several weeks. You've had a few interviews but haven't received a job offer. You're beginning to think it is hopeless, and you will never get a job. When you go on interviews, you feel nervous before and during because you continually think about how you are going to mess it up. You imagine the negative ways your interviewer is judging you. You know you should continue looking for a job, but your mind focuses on how tedious and frustrating the job search is. Instead of checking for new jobs, you procrastinate by watching television or check Facebook or Instagram. You feel worthless.

It is easy to blame your negative mood on the fact that you are jobless. But not having a job isn't a problem. It is your interpretation of your current and future situation that causes your mood and behavior.

**Scenario 2:** Imagine you have been looking for a job for several weeks. You have friends who spent months looking before they found their current positions. You decide to forego searching on job boards for today. Instead, you write a list of people you know who might be able to help. You reach out and ask them for contacts of people who might be hiring. You ask for tips to improve your interview skills. You remind yourself that every interview is an opportunity to practice. Every time you go on an interview, you remind yourself that you have the skills to make yourself successful in the job. After each meeting, you write down what went right and what you think you could improve for the next interview. With each conversation, you feel your confidence rise. You remain hopeful and motivated.

In both situations, you are unemployed. The difference is your view of yourself, others, and your expectations of the outcome. These different thought processes result in changed behavior and emotional reactions. In the first scenario, you view the situation with negative beliefs and thoughts, leading to adverse action (procrastination and avoiding the job search) and a negative mood (hopelessness and depression).

In the second approach, you focus on realistic outcomes and problem solving, which leads to effective behavior (continuing to look for a job) and a positive mood (hopefulness and motivation). The situation is a trigger to your thoughts, which leads to your behaviors and feelings.

**Perspective 1:** While you might think your unsuccessful job search causes your feelings of hopelessness, your belief that you won't succeed leads to procrastination and despair.

**Perspective 2:** Your interpretation of the job search, assuming your success, creates a more positive attitude and fosters continued motivation.

## Your Turn: What Kind of Thinker Are You?

What kind of thinker are you? What is your immediate reaction to stressful events and situations? Think of something you worry about (or something you worried about in the past). Be specific. Write down your primary concerns. The following examples are concerns you might have based on the previous scenarios:

**Perspective 1:** I'm concerned I won't get a job before depleting my savings. I am worried people will think I'm a loser. I am afraid that the longer I remain unemployed, the more I will be considered "unhirable."

**Perspective 2:** I'm concerned I won't get a job before dipping into my savings. I'm concerned my former colleagues will think I made a mistake for quitting my last job before having a secure position. I'm concerned the longer I stay unemployed, the harder it will be to get a new job.

Now look at your concerns and ask yourself: What is the worst possible outcome? The best? What is the most realistic result?

**Worst outcome:** Do not get a job and deplete savings.

**Best outcome:** Get the job of my dreams that recovers any savings I used.

**Realistic outcome:** Get a position that is better than my last job with a reasonable salary.

Which result does your list most resemble? Your answer reflects how you automatically think about stressful situations. If your primary concern doesn't match the most realistic outcome, go back and alter it to reflect the most realistic result. Then think about what behaviors and feelings might accompany this outcome.

When you worry about something, it helps to see different possibilities. It also helps to understand how your concerns compare to the most realistic outcomes. The next time you worry about something, list your worst, best, and most realistic results to help clarify your thinking.

## Seven Myths You Might Believe About CBT

Before we delve more into CBT and how it could work for you, let's look at some of the myths you might believe about it.

*Myth 1: CBT is just about positive thinking.*

One of the main aspects of CBT is to challenge negative beliefs; however, the premise is to replace these beliefs with realistic assumptions. If you currently have the idea that you are unlikeable, CBT doesn't work by simply replacing that belief with "I am likable." Instead, it works to find evidence in your life to challenge it; for example, if you have or have had friends, they probably liked you; therefore, you can't be unlikeable.

*Myth 2: CBT ignores emotions.*

Emotions are an integral part of CBT. The focus is on the connection between thoughts and feelings and the relationship between behavior and emotion. By changing your thought process and/or your actions, you can change how you feel about something.

*Myth 3: You never examine or consider childhood experiences in CBT.*

Indeed, CBT focuses more on the problems you are currently facing, but that doesn't mean that you never acknowledge your past. When working on core beliefs, it is crucial to understand where these beliefs came from to challenge them.

*Myth 4: There are too many structures in CBT, and it does not take the individual into consideration.*

There is a great deal of structure to CBT. There are basic outlines to how therapy should proceed and what should occur in a session; however, the uniqueness of the individual guides the therapist in determining which strategies and techniques work best.

*Myth 5: CBT only works on the surface and doesn't help resolve underlying issues.*

Understanding core beliefs is a necessary part of CBT. Core beliefs are deep-seated beliefs about yourself that often began in childhood. The theory behind CBT is that as you change your thinking and your behavior, you chip away at the distorted or untrue beliefs. Traditional psychoanalysis therapy works from the past to the present. CBT does the opposite. It starts with the present day, so you can change your perception and understanding of the past.

*Myth 6: Anxiety and depression are the only conditions helped by CBT.*

CBT, initially developed for use in the treatment of depression, is used today for anxiety, stress reduction, attention-deficit/hyperactivity disorder (ADHD), eating disorders, anger management, and grief; and CBT is used for management of physical conditions, such as chronic pain, menopause, heart disease, and insomnia.

*Myth 7: CBT is not effective in the long term.*

Numerous studies found that CBT is effective long term, partially because you can continue to use the tools and techniques throughout your life. The strategies used are transferable to many aspects of a person's life; for example, the same approach for changing a thought process for depression can help reduce stress.

# The Theory Behind CBT

CBT examines the relationship between your thoughts and behaviors. It focuses on how you think about yourself, the world, and other people. It works on the premise that most emotional and behavioral reactions are learned and, therefore, can be unlearned and replaced with a new way of reacting. CBT provides structure and tools to help, but the aim is to get you to a point you can "do it yourself" and work out your way of coping with problems. Some people describe CBT as guided self-help.

Some forms of psychotherapy focus on childhood experiences and how they influence your adult life. In contrast, CBT focuses on current problems, creates goals for overcoming those problems, and gives you step-by-step tools to help change your perspective—thereby improving your behavior and mood.

CBT empowers you to be in control by giving you a choice between negative and positive thoughts. It provides you with a set of tools to make choices. For example, instead of being emotionally overwhelmed, you can choose to be rational and create thoughts that are focused on coping and finding solutions. Rational thoughts are those based on facts and require the use of logical reasoning.

As you go through the CBT process in this book, try to practice the exercises consistently. In CBT, this is called *reality testing*. During reality testing, you assume your original negative thoughts are guesses as to what is happening or what might happen. Rather than seeing your first perspective as an accurate prediction, you test out other possibilities.

A big part of CBT is learning to gather evidence that contradicts biases in your thinking. Some of this reality testing involves using behavioral experiments to challenge your predictions and perspectives.

In keeping with the example about being unemployed, the assumption in your negative thoughts might include, "I will never get a job again, I will be unable to pay my rent, and my family will be homeless." Reality testing asks you to think about facts and then apply reasoning based on realistic values and outcomes. For example, you might think about how long it took you to get a job previously, how long it has taken others in your field to find a new job, what the current job market is like, and how much money you have in savings.

CBT reality testing might have you challenge the assumption "I am not worthwhile" by asking you to pay attention to specific areas of life where you have succeeded. It might have you question your thoughts of being a "failure" by asking you to complete an experiment where you readily see yourself as "successful." In the previous example, this could be securing at least one interview in the next week or successfully adding a new contact to your network.

CBT involves a specific set of steps:

1. Identify trigger events and conditions, such as grief, anger, depression, or anxiety.
2. Raise awareness of your reactions to these triggers, including thoughts, beliefs, emotions, and behaviors. Observe how you interpret the situations and events in your life.
3. Pinpoint harmful and inaccurate thoughts and beliefs.
4. Identify the physical, emotional, and behavioral responses that come along with these negative and inaccurate thoughts.
5. Set behavioral and emotional goals for how you want to react to these triggers.
6. Reality tests check the accuracy of your thinking by determining if you based your thoughts on facts or inaccurate perceptions.
7. Create new thoughts and attitudes about stressful triggers.
8. Practice implementing these new attitudes, behaviors, and emotions. Learn to integrate them into your life as new habits.

There will be times, especially at the beginning, when you feel uncomfortable or find the process painful. Changing long-standing beliefs about yourself, others, and the world around you is sometimes a complicated process. However, as you work through and practice each step, more helpful thinking and behavior will emerge. The exercises in this book help you work through these steps.

## Your Turn: Learning Your ABCs

The ABC chart is the staple of CBT, which is used to help identify negative thought processes. When you complete an ABC chart, you build awareness of how you think and reveal patterns of negative and irrational thinking. Also, it enables you to see how your thoughts affect your behaviors and emotions. The ABC chart can help you stop seeing the trigger as the cause of your reactions and understand that it is your thoughts (your interpretation) that cause your reaction.

**A** stands for *Activating Event* ("the trigger")

**B** stands for *Belief* or Thought

**C** stands for *Consequence* (behavioral and emotional)

To create an ABC chart, make three columns. Label them A, B, and C.

| A: Activating Event | B: Belief or Thought | C: Consequence |
|---|---|---|
| I need to give a speech. | I am going to make a fool of myself. I will forget everything I want to say, and everyone will think I'm stupid. I need to do well, or else…. | I feel anxious. My stomach hurts. I can't sleep. I can't focus. |
| I didn't get the promotion at work. | I deserved that promotion. I can't believe they treated me with such disrespect. My boss never liked me. I work harder than anyone else. Hard work is what it's about; this is just unfair. | I feel angry. I'm not going to try at work anymore. I'm going to tell my boss what I think of him. |
| I didn't get the job. | I need a job. The interviewer is judging me. I'll never get a job. | I feel sad because I'm never going to get a job. I should just quit looking. |

If you are having difficulty completing your chart, try working backward. Start with the consequence—what you feel and your behavior. Then consider why you feel that way and what happened to bring on those thoughts.

This chart is a primary CBT tool and one we'll return to often in this book, sometimes adding additional columns to help you understand and challenge your thoughts.

## Understanding Themes

All feelings have related themes in your thoughts. Here's a quick tip sheet to help you identify thoughts that drive your emotions.

**Anger/frustration:** I perceive an obstacle threatening me in some way. The constraint can be something from the past, present, or future.

**Anxiety/nervousness:** I perceive a threat that will harm me or challenge my security. The danger can be from the present or future.

**Sadness/disappointment:** I perceive a loss. I won't be entirely satisfied as a result. The loss can be from the past, present, or anticipated in the future.

**Excitement/happiness:** I perceive receiving something that enhances my life situation. It can be from the past, present, or future anticipation.

**Shame/embarrassment:** I perceive that I am responsible for some wrongdoing toward others or myself.

## Benefits of CBT

Numerous research studies show CBT is as effective as medicine in treating disorders such as depression and anxiety. Because CBT teaches skills used even after treatment has ended, it can be more effective than medication. Some of the distinct advantages of this type of therapy include the following:

**Short term.** When working with a therapist, the average number of CBT sessions is 16. It is a closed-end treatment; unlike traditional therapy, it does not continue indefinitely.

**Targeted.** CBT teaches specific skills and corrects negative and problematic thinking processes. Once you understand how to use these skills, you "get better."

**Structured.** CBT includes specific tools, techniques, strategies, and steps.

**Instructive.** Whether you work with a therapist or use exercises in this book on your own, you learn to cope with stress and other problems in your life constructively, so you can counsel yourself.

**Adaptive.** You can use CBT strategies in many different situations. You might have chosen to use CBT to overcome a fear of dogs or to manage your anger. However, once you learn to use the techniques, you can employ them in other areas of your everyday life.

**Measurable.** CBT works with specific goals—for example, overcoming your fear of flying—and has specific steps for reaching your goal. Because of this, you can see and measure your progress along the way.

CBT is one of the most extensively studied forms of psychotherapy, with hundreds of published studies. A 2005 review of studies showed it to be highly effective in treating depression, generalized anxiety disorder, panic disorder, social phobia, and post-traumatic stress disorder.

As you continue to use CBT and the techniques become habitual, you might notice an improvement in many areas of your life. Your relationships become more fulfilling, your problem-solving skills improve, your self-esteem increases, and you feel greater overall satisfaction with life.

## Disadvantages of CBT

As with all treatments, CBT has its share of proponents and critics. Some critics worry that because CBT focuses so much on current problems, it doesn't adequately address underlying issues, such as childhood abuse and doesn't help you resolve your feelings toward those. It is also an individual treatment and doesn't always address family issues or interpersonal relationships.

There aren't many risks to using CBT. As discussed earlier in the chapter, you might feel uncomfortable or discouraged at first when facing long-held views of the world, your environment, and yourself. There might be times when you cry or feel angry and emotionally drained. You might feel anxious, such as when you are confronting fears. However, as you work through the exercises in this book, the discomfort should lessen. And as you learn new coping skills, you can better deal with fears and negative thought patterns.

CBT takes commitment. With CBT, you need to complete exercises and train yourself to think in different ways. It takes time, energy, and practice to bring about positive change. There aren't instant results with CBT.

## Comparing CBT to Other Forms of Therapy

CBT is one type of therapy, but there are others you might find useful. The following are brief descriptions of some of the main types of treatments.

*Psychoanalysis* is a long-term form of therapy and is what most people think of when they hear the term *psychological therapy*. It is an in-depth talk therapy geared toward bringing unconscious or buried thoughts and feelings to the conscious mind so they can be examined and resolved. Working on repressed emotions and experiences from childhood are often part of the therapy process.

*Psychodynamic therapy* is short term; often, present-day actions and behaviors can be influenced by about 15-16 sessions that are meant to increase self-awareness of past experiences. During sessions, the therapist works with you to examine past unresolved conflicts and dysfunctional relationships to determine patterns in emotions and thoughts to better cope with problems in your present-day life. It can help with depression, anxiety disorders, personality disorders, stress, and other mental illnesses.

*Acceptance and commitment therapy (ACT)* focuses on developing an acceptance of intense emotional feelings as a normal reaction to past events, such as traumatic events, physical illness, or problematic relationships. Acknowledging and accepting these feelings allow you to continue moving forward and making changes in behavior to live a fulfilling life. ACT has been found effective in treating numerous conditions, including workplace stress, social anxiety disorder, depression, and obsessive-compulsive disorder.

Each type of therapy has benefits and disadvantages. CBT is a prevalent form of treatment, possibly because it is easily accessible. Not only do many therapists work with CBT, but there are also many online self-help courses and apps that have brought CBT into the public eye over the past decade.

# Your Turn: Is CBT Right for Me?

CBT works for many different conditions and situations, but that doesn't mean it is right for you. The following checklist covers some of the health conditions and circumstances where CBT can help. Check all that apply to you.

- [x] Anger problems
- [x] Anxiety
- [ ] Body dysmorphic disorder
- [ ] Chronic fatigue
- [ ] Chronic pain
- [x] Depression
- [ ] Eating disorders (such as anorexia or bulimia)
- [ ] Gambling
- [x] Guilt and shame
- [ ] Hoarding
- [x] Low self-esteem
- [ ] Obsessive-compulsive disorder
- [x] Panic attacks
- [x] Performance anxiety
- [ ] Personality disorder
- [ ] Post-traumatic stress disorder
- [x] Sexual or relationship problems
- [x] Sleep problems
- [ ] Social phobia
- [x] Specific phobias (such as fear of flying or dogs)
- [x] Spending money excessively
- [x] Stress
- [ ] Substance abuse
- [x] Worrying

You might have checked more than one area, as problems tend to overlap. Don't worry; it is common to have more than one area that needs improvement. As you use CBT strategies, you might find secondary problems improve as well.

In addition to identifying specific issues, there are other considerations before beginning CBT. This type of therapy is solution-oriented, not talk-oriented. Even when you work with a therapist, there is less emphasis on talking about how your week was and there is more focus on learning and practicing how to process your triggers differently. However, some people find they want someone to listen. Consider the following CBT Readiness Quiz and check those that apply to you.

**CBT Readiness Quiz:**
- [x] 1. I am ready to make a positive change in my life.
- [x] 2. There are practical problems, such as sleep problems, anxiety, anger, or depression, that I would like to improve.
- [x] 3. I am willing to commit time each week to complete exercises.
- [x] 4. I have a support system of friends and family.
- [x] 5. I can work independently, or I can use this book with my therapist.
- [x] 6. I don't want to keep dwelling on the past; I would like to solve problems in my present and future life.
- [x] 7. I need to deal with issues before focusing on specific areas to improve.
- [ ] 8. I don't know what I want to improve; I just know I don't like my life.
- [ ] 9. I don't know if I have the time to complete the exercises right now.
- [ ] 10. I am alone and feel that this might stir up too much emotion.
- [x] 11. I think I need the help of a therapist to work on the exercises and want someone who will listen to my problems.
- [ ] 12. I have unresolved issues from my past I think should be addressed.

If you checked items in numbers 1 through 6, you are ready to delve into CBT and make it work for you. If you checked more items in numbers 7 through 12, you might want to consider working with a CBT therapist and using this book as a tool.

CBT is an effective strategy for dealing with many conditions and situations, such as depression, anxiety, anger, and relationships. It empowers you to choose positive thinking over negative thinking patterns, based on the premise that your thoughts lead to feelings, which influence actions. The skills you learn in CBT can be carried over to many aspects of your life.

# CHAPTER 2
# Interpreting Your Thoughts and Feelings

Are your thoughts a result of your feelings? Or are your feelings a result of your thoughts? It is essential to understand not only which causes which, but how to separate thoughts from feelings. In Chapter 1, you learned how thoughts create feelings and behaviors. In this chapter, you'll learn how feelings sometimes lead to unhealthy thought patterns. The exercises help you move from reasoning based on emotions to reasoning based on your thoughts. We look at some common unhealthy thought patterns and provide strategies for looking at situations in your life more helpfully.

## Thoughts, Feelings, and Behaviors

Thoughts, feelings, and behaviors work together in a continuous cycle. First, you have a thought, which influences how you feel and behave. You then have thoughts about those feelings and actions, which affect how you think and behave. The cycle continues.

Imagine you are at a party where you don't know anyone except the host. As you make your way around the room, you spot a familiar face but cannot recall the person's name. You recognize her as someone who used to sit near you to at work but you haven't seen since you left the company a few years back. You begin to feel nervous, thinking, "I am embarrassed that I don't remember her name. It would be awkward to talk to her and admit I don't remember her name. I should avoid her." And with that, you walk in the opposite direction. Your inner voice validates your actions. "We were never friends at work. I wouldn't have much to say to her." You feel relieved.

You might believe you felt nervous because you couldn't remember your coworker's name and that you walked away because you felt shy. But it wasn't the situation that causes your feelings, and it wasn't your feelings that caused you to walk away; it was your perception that caused your feelings and actions. Your initial thoughts drove how you felt and probably came so quickly that you were unaware of them until you felt anxious, but they were present the entire time.

Maybe you were so focused on your nervousness that you didn't notice your immediate thoughts.

You might have thought the following:

- I should only approach people I know well.
- I am stupid because I can't remember her name.
- I shouldn't put myself into embarrassing situations.
- The people she is talking to will judge me.
- People I don't know well are intimidating.

These underlying thoughts created a feeling of nervousness, and then that feeling spurred your action—avoiding her for the rest of the night so you wouldn't have to feel uncomfortable. This anxious feeling also influenced your thoughts for the remainder of the party. You became self-conscious and thought that other people were judging you and that you didn't fit in. These thoughts spiraled into feelings of despair, which made you feel like a failure.

In this example, you allowed your emotions to control your thoughts and, therefore, to control your actions. Your reasoning and self-talk revolved around how you felt. *Self-talk* refers to running commentary in your mind, the voice in your head that reflects and interprets the world around you. When you make a conscious decision to change your self-talk into a more positive view of the situation, you change your response.

Using the ABC chart described in Chapter 1, the party scenario looks like this:

| A: Activating Event | B: Belief or Thought | C: Consequences |
| --- | --- | --- |
| I see someone who looks familiar. | I don't know her well enough to approach. | Embarrassment |
| | | Nervousness |
| | I am pathetic because I can't remember her name. | Look away and avoid her |
| | Talking to people I don't know well is intimidating. | |
| I feel uncomfortable and nervous. | I can't handle feeling uncomfortable. | Nervousness |
| | | Avoidance |
| My hands are shaking. | My nervousness will show, and everyone will judge me. | Leave party |
| My heart is racing. | | |

# Chapter 2: Interpreting Your Thoughts and Feelings

From this table, you see that your original thoughts and feelings led to a new activating event and, therefore, a new set of emotions and behaviors. By stopping, examining your thoughts, and coming up with alternative beliefs, you change your perception of the situation and your reactions.

You can add two additional columns to the chart to incorporate this new information:

**D:** New Beliefs

**E:** New Consequences

Your new beliefs are ways of combating your immediate reaction. It takes practice to notice these thoughts, analyze them, and come up with a more helpful and healthy way of looking at the situation. The following table provides examples of new alternative thoughts and shows how your behaviors change once you look at the situation with a fresh perspective.

| A: Activating Event | B: Belief or Thought | C: Consequences | D: New Beliefs | E: New Consequences |
|---|---|---|---|---|
| I see someone I used to work with but can't remember her name. | She will judge me. She will be upset that I don't know her name. It's my fault that I didn't keep in touch with her. I should only talk to people I know well. I can't handle feeling uncomfortable; it's a sign I should avoid her. | Nervousness Self-blame Avoid her Leave party | I don't need to know everyone well to say, "Hi." This is an opportunity to get to know her better. She is just as guilty of not keeping in touch. Her judgments are harmless. | I am feeling more relaxed. A little nervous but not too uncomfortable. Approach her and catch up. |
| I feel uncomfortable. My hand is shaking. My heart is racing a bit. | I can't handle feeling uncomfortable. Feeling uncomfortable is a sign I should avoid her. She will judge my nervousness. | Nervousness Self-blame Avoid her Leave party | I don't have to let my uncomfortable feelings run my life. I can take a few deep breaths and calm down. | I am feeling more confident. She is probably nervous, too. I can approach her. |

## Your Turn: New Beliefs

In Chapter 1, you created an ABC chart listing some of your worries. Use this chart and add columns D (New Beliefs) and E (New Consequences). Try to come up with new ways of looking at the situation, and imagine how your behavior changes with a fresh perspective.

Over the next week, keep track of times you feel stressed or upset. Complete the ABCDE chart, trying to come up with an alternative or new belief, and think about what new consequences could occur.

Completing this exercise helps open your mind to new beliefs or at least the possibility of a different way of viewing the situation. In the beginning, you might not believe all the new beliefs you write down. That's okay. Work on carrying out the new behaviors anyway. As you do, you will begin to accept the views.

## Separating Thoughts from Emotions

By now, you should understand that your thoughts drive your emotions, and by changing what you think, you can change how you feel. You can make a conscious decision to review your thinking process and make a conscious decision to change it when needed.

There might be times you find separating your thoughts from your emotions is complicated and confusing. It is often helpful to work backward. First, consider how you feel and then think about what happened (the triggering event) to invoke those feelings. For example, "I'm feeling hurt and angry. Jordan said he would text at 7 P.M. and didn't." You identified your feelings and the triggering event.

Now, consider the thoughts you had as a result. You might have thought, "I am not important to Jordan." Try changing this thought to, "Jordan is my friend. I am sure he will text when he gets a chance. Something must have come up." This thought brings up a completely different reaction than believing you are not important. Instead of feeling hurt and angry, you are calm and confident that your relationship is healthy.

Creating a new thought is the easy part, believing it is a different story. You can tell yourself that Jordan is your friend and will text when available, but you might be fighting other thoughts—the ones that tell you he doesn't care, he found someone else to go to dinner with, or that he simply blew you off. Continue repeating the new thought, "Jordan is my friend; he will text when available." When your mind returns to the original view, consciously replace it with the new one. Remember, you get to choose your thoughts; you get to decide how you feel.

Often, we place the blame for our feelings on someone or something else. You might think that it is Jordan who made you hurt and angry, but that is wrong. It is your perception of the event—I am not important to Jordan—that caused your hurt and anger. Learning to separate your thoughts and emotions gives you control of how you feel and react.

Mixing up emotions and thoughts frequently leads to a cycle of negative thinking. Your first thought, "I am not important to Jordan," starts your mind on a search for events to justify this belief. You remember that last week, he was late when meeting for lunch. You think about the time he said he didn't have time to meet up with you. You think about the time he brushed off your opinion as not relevant. The more you think about it, the more you are convinced that you are right—Jordan doesn't care. Instead of separating your thoughts and emotions, you allow your emotions to drive your thoughts.

Avoidance is another typical example of a negative, emotion-driven thought process. Typically, the more you avoid something, the more you fear it. Imagine you are afraid of flying. You avoid getting on a plane because the anxiousness makes you uncomfortable. You limit where you go to places you can drive. Using the ABC method, the following shows how negative thinking patterns lead to more negative thinking.

**A:** I need to get on an airplane.

**B:** It is scary to fly. It makes me anxious and uncomfortable, and I can't handle the discomfort.

**C:** The best thing to do is always to avoid flying by canceling the trip or driving.

Once you decided to avoid the plane trip, you feel relieved. You have avoided the discomfort of being nervous, which internalizes and reinforces your negative thinking. You believe you should always avoid flying, but you might also think that there is something wrong with you; you might think that you should be able to get over your fear, but you can't, so you are defective.

Now, imagine you make decisions based on your thoughts instead of allowing your emotions to control both your thoughts and actions:

**Original B:** It is scary to fly. It makes me anxious and uncomfortable, and I can't handle the discomfort.

**Alternative B:** I can handle the discomfort. I can do deep breathing when I am on the plane and remember that the flight will end, and I will be back on the ground in a few hours.

**Original C:** The best thing to do is always to avoid flying by canceling the trip or driving.

**Alternative C:** The more I fly, the easier it will get. I can overcome my discomforts.

As you see, negative thinking usually causes more negative thinking. It becomes a cycle; you think a negative thought and feel and react negatively. You then are irritable, which causes more negative thoughts, which worsens your mood, which creates even more negative thoughts. The following section examines some common negative thinking patterns and provides questions you can ask yourself to combat the thought processes.

# Problematic Thought Processes

If you think something often enough, you believe it is true. If you think in the same way often enough, it becomes a habit, even if it is unhelpful. We use cognitive distortions to convince us of something that isn't true or to justify our feelings and actions. Cognitive distortions are biased habits in the way you think. They cause overly rigid and negative thoughts. It's like wearing rose-colored glasses and assuming everything is a shade of pink.

For example, if you tell yourself you will fail anytime you try something new, you justify not trying new things. This is seeing things in absolutes—one type of problematic thought pattern. There are different types of cognitive distortions.

## Catastrophizing

When you catastrophize, you magnify every problem and assume everything is going to end in a colossal disaster. You believe your imagined outcome is a given, and you don't see how it could turn out well. You fail to take steps to prevent a problem because you can't change the result.

Examples:

- You argue with your boyfriend and assume you will break up.
- You make a small mistake at work and assume you will get fired.

Questions to ask yourself:

- What evidence do I have to prove or disprove my conclusion?
- How likely is this to happen?
- What are the other possible outcomes?

## Mind Reading

When you engage in mind reading, you guess what other people are thinking and assume it is true. You automatically believe others have a negative opinion of you and become angry, anxious, or depressed because of these assumptions. You act as though your ideas are correct without any evidence.

Examples:

- You see a negative post about someone's actions on Facebook, assume it is about you, and send a mean private message.
- You see someone on the street you recently met. He ignores you, and you assume he doesn't want to talk to you.

Questions to ask yourself:

- What are some alternative explanations?
- How can I test my guess?

## Fortune-Telling

Fortune-telling is a thought pattern in which you make predictions, usually with a negative outcome, and then you feel discouraged or behave based on a reality that hasn't yet happened and might never happen.

Examples:

- You want to get to know someone better but assume she won't want to meet you, so you never bother trying to talk to her.
- Your boss asks to speak to you about your work, and you assume you are getting fired, so you avoid the conversation as long as possible.

Questions to ask yourself:

- What would happen if I take the risk and do it anyway?
- What else might happen?
- If the negative does happen, what steps can I take to deal with it?

## Black-and-White Thinking

When you think in terms of black and white, you categorize outcomes and assume things are either good or bad. You don't see any middle ground. Your bad category is extensive and includes most results; your good outcomes are limited.

Examples:

- Your daughter applies to 10 colleges but has a clear preference. You assume any school other than her first choice will be socially and scholastically awful for her.
- You try a new sport, and when you aren't the best on the team, you believe you are a failure. You stop playing.
- Your friend invites someone else to an event. You assume she is no longer your friend and stop reaching out.

Questions to ask yourself:

- Is there a middle ground I am ignoring?
- Am I imposing superhuman qualities on myself?
- What is the evidence for and against this thinking?

## Overgeneralizing

When you overgeneralize, you assume that what happened once will always occur, and something that didn't happen never will. You see problems as never ending and hopeless. You use the words "always" or "never" to describe specific situations. You ignore exceptions and focus on global results. You assume that a poor outcome in the past indicates it will always end that way.

Examples:

- You think, "I always mess up."
- You think, "I can't trust anyone."
- You didn't get a promotion and believe you never will.
- It rains on the day you planned a picnic, and your first reaction is, "It always rains when I plan something outdoors."

Questions to ask yourself:

- Am I attributing too much importance to a one-time event?
- Are there parts that I can control in the future?
- Are there past events I am ignoring?
- Do I need everything to go my way?

Success comes from investing in a situation, even if it is not ideal. By assuming the ship that sailed without you was the only and best ship leaves you feeling stranded and alone. Think about one time you did not get what you wanted in life. Did you stop there and assume there were no other options? Or did you continue and look for something equally good or better?

## Personalization and Blame

Thought patterns of personalization and blame happen when you take responsibility for events out of your control or blame others for events in your control. You make up things that have nothing to do with you about you.

Examples:

- The Uber driver goes down a street where there is a detour. You assume he is trying to take advantage of you by driving up the cost.
- You make plans with a friend and then need to cancel. When your friend seems disappointed, you assume he is mad at you rather than merely disappointed.
- Your spouse forgets your anniversary. You think it was on purpose because you forgot to celebrate the promotion she received a month ago.

Questions to ask yourself:

- What are other factors that contributed to the situation?
- What factors are your responsibility? Where do you have control?
- If someone is upset, is she upset with me or with the situation?

## Ignoring the Positive

When you ignore the positive, you look at the negative aspects of a situation. You discredit positive information or turn it around to be negative. You filter information and use only the information that supports your contrary view. You believe life is unfair.

Examples:

- You don't get a job; you assume it was a perfect position and discount the idea that there might be a position that is a better fit.
- A coworker asks if you want to go to lunch; you assume he asked because no one else was around.
- A friend asks you for a favor. You think, "Now I know why we are friends; he just wants to use me."

Questions to ask yourself:

- What are the positive elements of the situation?
- What information am I forgetting?
- Is there a possible "silver lining"?

According to the American Psychological Association, people who see the glass as "half full" are healthier. They live longer, have lower rates of depression, don't catch colds as often, have a reduced risk of dying from cardiovascular disease, and rate their emotional well-being higher than those who have a negative view of life.

## "Should" and "Must"

When you think in absolutes, you have strong beliefs and rules about how other people should act and become angry when they don't behave that way. You make demands on the behavior of others. You use "should" statements on yourself, "I should have done that," and you feel guilty for what you did or didn't do.

Examples:

- A cashier is abrupt and rude. You become angry because "People must treat me with respect."
- Your spouse comes home late. You are angry because she should call if she is running late.
- You are upset because you can't find your keys. You believe you should always be responsible and hang them on the hook when you come home.

Questions to ask yourself:

- Are there exceptions to this rule? What circumstances could allow for flexibility?
- Why do other people need to live by my rules?
- Does this person have different beliefs or priorities that compete with my ideas of how she should act?

Distorted thinking quickly causes you to categorize requests about your behavior or the behavior of others as demands rather than as a statement of preference or desire. This causes unnecessary defensiveness and negative emotions. Over the next week, practice viewing all requests as statements of choice rather than impositions by changing "should" or "must" to "I prefer."

## Emotional Reasoning

When you use emotional reasoning, you base conclusions about yourself, others, and the world on your feelings. You assume that if you feel something, it must be true.

Examples:

- "I feel angry with you, so you must have done something wrong or tried to take advantage of me."
- You feel guilty and assume you must have done something terrible.
- You feel overwhelmed. You assume your problems are insurmountable.

Questions to ask yourself:

- What are the thoughts behind my emotions?
- When I remove the emotion, what are the facts?

## Labeling

When you engage in labeling, you label your behavior and the behavior of others in a negative way, such as "I am stupid" or "He is lazy."

Examples:

- Your brother-in-law has a hard time finding a job. You think he is lazy.
- You made a mistake at work; you think you are a loser.

Questions to ask yourself:

- How can I state this by focusing on specific actions without making personal attacks?
- What are some positive traits in myself and others?

# Your Turn: Notice Your Thoughts

Use the ABC worksheet introduced in Chapter 1. See if you spot the distortion type for each thought or set of thoughts. Don't worry about doing it right or wrong. The point is to begin to develop an awareness of your biases in thinking and notice your habits.

**Situation:** You are at a party and see someone you recognize but don't know well. You are afraid to go up and speak to him.

**Thought:** I don't know him well; I shouldn't bother him.

**Distortion:** "Should" statement. You are applying an internal rule that limits your behavior.

**Situation:** You are having a hard day. You text a friend, but she doesn't respond.

**Thought:** She is never around when I need her.

**Distortion:** Overgeneralization. You used the word "never" when she previously responded to your texts.

**Situation:** You go to the store for butter. You come home with milk and bread but forgot the butter.

**Thought**: I am such an idiot. Why didn't I write down what I wanted to buy?

**Distortion:** Labeling. You labeled your forgetfulness as a negative attribute.

Pay attention to your thoughts and use the same format to determine what types of problematic thinking processes you use.

When you first start CBT and begin working on the exercises in this book, it might not be possible to sit down and work through your thoughts. Or you might not be able to catch your negative thought patterns and work through them in your mind. Use a notebook or an app on your phone or tablet to log the situation and what you are thinking. Later when you have time, you can analyze your thoughts and actions and what might have been different if you had thought more healthily.

Your thoughts influence your feelings and behaviors. One of the core tenets of CBT is by changing your thought process, you change how you feel and act. There are numerous problematic thought processes, and most people tend to use the same ones repeatedly. When you understand your thinking patterns, you can modify your thoughts and make them more helpful.

# CHAPTER 3
# Automatic Thoughts, Assumptions, and Core Beliefs

You interpret the world around you instantly and without any conscious effort. As you go through the day, thoughts pop into your mind, telling you how to feel and how to react. Sometimes, you are aware of these thoughts; sometimes, you are not. You might not even realize this is happening because the idea occurs in a split second. Suppose you run into a friend you haven't seen in years. Your mind instantly brings up fun memories, and you feel happy and excited. You probably focus more on the happiness emotion than you do on the fleeting thoughts. You might believe seeing your old friend caused your joy, but your interpretation of the event—your memories or thoughts of fun times—caused you to feel happy.

## Your First Reaction

Remember, it isn't the event itself that creates emotions; instead, it's your interpretation of the event that creates emotions. The immediate thoughts you have—the ones that occur spontaneously and without your consent—are called *automatic thoughts*. You don't plan automatic thoughts, and you don't spend time thinking them through. Often, you don't even realize you had a thought. Automatic thoughts reflect how you see yourself, other people, and the world around you.

Automatic thoughts can be positive, negative, or neutral, depending on your view of the situation. If you see someone you recognize, your thoughts might be…

*Positive:* I remember her from Barbara's birthday party. We had a friendly conversation.

*Negative:* I recognize her, but I don't remember her name. I am so stupid.

*Neutral:* I recognize her, but I can't remember her name.

In this book, we mostly address positive and negative thoughts; however, you should know that they can sometimes be neutral.

As you worked through the exercises in Chapter 2, you learned to separate your emotions from your immediate reaction—your automatic thoughts. You accept that these thoughts drive your feelings. Even though they happen in an instant, you can learn to listen to, label, and then dispute your automatic thoughts and, therefore, change how you see yourself, others, and the world around you.

## Your Turn: Listening to Self-Talk

Close your eyes. Imagine an event where you had a mildly adverse reaction. Visualize the scenario in your mind. As you replay the scene, try to connect with the emotion you feel and listen to what you say to yourself.

Jot down your thoughts.

This exercise helps you develop the ability to connect to your inner voice. As you continue to practice, you will be more in tune with your inner voice as a situation unfolds rather than having to look back later.

## Negative Automatic Thoughts

Negative automatic thoughts often reflect a poor self-image, a sour or vulnerable view of your environment, or a belief that a situation will turn out poorly. These types of thoughts usually lead to negative emotions, such as anger, anxiety, sadness, or guilt.

Some examples of negative automatic thoughts:

- I am ugly; I will always be lonely.
- I overslept. I am such an idiot. Now I am going to get fired.
- Tom is very irritable today. What did I do to cause his bad mood?
- This project is hard. I'll never get it done. I can't do anything right.
- I argued with my partner. All my relationships fail. Why bother trying?
- I don't want to speak at the meeting; I always sound stupid.
- I didn't call Charlie back; he must think I am a terrible friend.
- That salesperson was rude. What did I do wrong?

When left to run rampant, your negative automatic thoughts affect your mood, self-esteem, and overall feelings of happiness. It is probably more comfortable and more believable for you to think negatively about yourself than to think positively, especially when these thoughts are a result of past events. For example, if you routinely refer to yourself as stupid, you might have heard this about yourself throughout your childhood. However, as an adult, you can consciously choose to change these to reflect a more positive and realistic view of yourself. Negative automatic thoughts tend to be self-fulfilling. If you tell yourself you are going to fail, you increase your chance of failing.

# Changing Negative Self-Talk

Learning to listen to your automatic thoughts is the first step toward changing them. Once you stop and hear what you tell yourself, you can challenge the idea, come up with an alternative view, and decide which thought you want to keep.

Suppose you are driving. You follow the speed limit and are cautious. The driver behind you is upset, beeping his horn when you don't quickly move after a light turns green. When you look in your rearview mirror, you can see him yelling at you. You immediately go back over the past several minutes. What did you do wrong? Why is this person angry at you? You must have done something to upset him.

You don't bother looking for other reasons why this person is upset that have nothing to do with you. For example:

- Maybe he is having a bad day.
- Maybe he was just fired.
- Maybe someone he knows went into the hospital, and he is impatient to get there.
- Maybe he is a jerk.

Many different reasons could have prompted his aggressive behavior that had nothing to do with you. By changing how you look at the situation, you change how you feel. At first, you blamed yourself for the other driver's actions and felt upset, guilty, or scared. When you look for other possible reasons for the behavior, you think differently. You might feel sympathetic because there is a reason this person is so upset. Your whole demeanor changes, and you pull over to let him pass, smiling and waving as he drives by.

Often, you base automatic thoughts on incomplete information and don't take time to analyze each thought that pops into your mind. Because you created them on past experiences and beliefs, they are believable; therefore, you see them as accurate even though they can be distorted or wrong. You might have utilized one of the problematic thought processes outlined in Chapter 2 to create the thought. In the previous example, you can see that personalization and blame were at play.

To have a more balanced and positive perspective, you need to stop, pay attention to your thoughts, dispute their validity if necessary, and reframe your thinking. One way to do that is to use your ABC chart. You can use the questions listed after each problematic thought pattern to start the process, and add your questions to the list. Keep in mind there are no right or wrong answers. The goal of answering the questions is to help you feel and manage problematic situations differently.

The following is an example of using a version of the ABC chart to aid you in challenging your immediate reaction:

| A: Situation | B: Belief or Thought | C: Behavior | D: Questions |
|---|---|---|---|
| You have plans to go away for a weekend with your spouse, and she wants to change weekends based on a work meeting. | This is unfair. She is selfish. Everything needs to be on her terms. She never communicates. She is trying to make me feel guilty for not being accepting of the change. | Yell. Give the silent treatment. Refuse to listen to her side. | Why did she change the dates? Is there something important going on at work that she feels she cannot miss? Are there other factors that contributed to the decision? Is there additional information I need to know? Can I take some responsibility for the lack of communication? How can I talk about this without making accusations and personal attacks? What are the facts? Can I separate my emotions from my reaction and look at the situation rationally? |

In this example, your immediate reaction is anger. You used several different problematic thought processes to arrive at angry. Read through Column B again, and try to identify personalization and blame, labeling, overgeneralizing, and emotional reasoning. Notice how the questions in Column D combat these unhealthy thinking processes. Your new perspective of the situation might be…

> *This was not meant to upset me. It was done based on changing priorities. We need to work together to find a solution.*

When you first found out about the change of dates, you were upset and angry. Now with a different perspective, you are ready to discuss the situation and find a solution.

## Your Turn: Questions to Ask Yourself

*The form accompanying this exercise is in Appendix C.*

Over the next week, as soon as you notice a negative emotion (anger, anxiety, sadness, and so on), write down five questions to ask yourself to challenge your thoughts.

Some examples of questions include the following:

- What emotion am I feeling?
- Does this emotion fit the situation?
- What thoughts did I have right before this emotion?
- What problematic thought process did I use?
- What additional information do I need to know?

## Making Assumptions

When you accept your ideas as accurate without having proof, you make assumptions. When you fail to ask for more information and don't look for evidence of a thought, you make assumptions. This leads to acting on unhealthy thinking processes and incomplete information. You act on assumptions, not facts.

*Some assumptions you make are valid.* For example, your dog is standing near the door barking. You assume he needs to go outside. Sometimes, assumptions help keep you safe. For example, you are visiting a city you have never been to and believe you should not walk the streets alone.

*Sometimes, assumptions can limit you.* For example, when you assume it is not safe to walk the streets alone when visiting a new city, you might decide you always need to stay inside the hotel. You limit your behavior based on an idea without having evidence to back it up. You could challenge your belief by finding solutions, such as asking the concierge or desk clerk what streets are safe to walk alone or calling an Uber.

*Some assumptions are unhelpful.* Suppose you text your partner, and for several hours, you don't receive a response. You continue to text, but still, there is no response. All afternoon, you assume something bad happened, or he is angry at you. You spend the day going back and forth between being worried there was an accident and being mad because he is ignoring you. These thoughts interfere with your job. Later, you find out he was working with a colleague on a project and left his phone in his desk drawer, you realize your assumptions were wrong, and you wasted your day believing untrue assumptions.

When you make assumptions, you…

- *Miss opportunities.* You want to ask someone on a date but are assume she will say no, so you never ask.
- *Make errors in judgments and decisions.* You assume you know a person's personality based on his appearance.
- *Misunderstand others.* You assume you know the reasons behind an action without asking.
- *Have a hard time deciding.* You imagine too many scenarios (mostly with adverse outcomes) and find it challenging to choose one.

Assumptions are stories you create to help you understand the people and the world around you. But these stories often have nothing to do with reality. Assumptions add to problems rather than creating solutions. You jump to a conclusion without having all the facts or the whole story. You make decisions based on incomplete information.

## Your Turn: Turning Assumptions Around

*The form accompanying this exercise is in Appendix C.*

There are six steps to turning assumptions around and reacting to the reality of the situation:

1. Write down the facts as you know them.
2. Write down the assumptions you are making.
3. Identify problematic thought processes.
4. Write down additional information as you know it.
5. Determine all possible actions you can take. Cross out those that rely on assumptions.
6. Select a response that uses facts.

The next time you find yourself assuming, stop assuming and follow the steps. Doing this ensures you don't act rashly based on incomplete information.

**Situation:** You are expecting a text from your friend Chris about meeting for dinner after work. It is almost time to leave, and you haven't heard anything.

**Step 1** Facts: You usually leave work around 5:00 p.m. It is 4:30, and Chris hasn't texted.

**Step 2** Assumptions:

- Chris doesn't want to have dinner with me.
- Chris decided to have dinner with someone else.

- Chris is ignoring me.
- Chris has been busy all day and hasn't had the chance to call or text.

**Step 3** Negative Thinking Patterns:

Fortune-telling—making an error in reasoning without knowing all the information and filling in the information you don't know with assumptions.

**Step 4** Extraneous Facts:

Chris told me about the big project at work.

**Step 5** Actions:

- Text Chris to see if we are still meeting for dinner.
- Run personal errands after work to give Chris extra time to get done.
- Eat at home, and meet Chris another night.

**Step 6:** Response:

I will text Chris. If I don't hear back before I leave, I will run some errands to give him additional time to answer.

We usually assume people think just like we do, without giving them credit for having their own thoughts and ideas. To stop making assumptions, accept that people think differently, and you shouldn't guess what they are thinking. Instead, ask and listen to their answers.

# Tips for Eliminating Assumptions

Just as you need to catch the automatic thoughts and make a conscious effort to change them, you can listen to your inner talk and learn not to make assumptions.

**Ask questions.** Ask questions to clarify what you think. Find out information about the situation or the person.

**Listen.** Practice active listening, which involves putting aside your assumptions to focus on what the other person is saying. Be present in the moment, and try repeating back their words to assure you heard them correctly.

**Give the benefit of the doubt.** When we jump to conclusions about someone else's behavior, we often assume negative motivations. When you give someone the benefit of the doubt, you attribute his actions to positive or neutral thoughts until you have information to the contrary.

**Consider the past.** Consider this person's actions and motivations from the past. For example, if Chris is typically reliable, why would you assume he is not this time?

**Resist stereotypes.** Placing a label on someone is assuming something about her character without any information. Prejudice about ethnicity, religion, gender, or appearance is assuming character traits without knowing anything about the person.

Ask yourself if you are making a rational decision based on facts or jumping to a conclusion. Ask yourself if you have enough information to make a judgment or a decision, or if you should gather additional information. Remember, no matter how long you have known someone, you can't know what he is thinking; it is always better to ask.

# Your Turn: Uncovering Your Assumptions

You base assumptions on unhelpful thinking processes, usually fortune-telling (making predictions without adequate information) or mind reading (believing you know what someone else is thinking). To discover when you most often jump to assumptions, complete the following sentence:

When I feel upset, I assume someone is...

- Going to reject me.
- Putting me in a vulnerable situation or taking advantage of me by_____.
- Going to say no to my request.
- Planning to criticize me.
- Going to hurt me emotionally or cause me pain.
- Angry with me.

Think back to a situation when you assumed something about another person. Was one of these reasons behind the assumption? If so, which one? If not, what caused you to jump to this conclusion?

Is there an assumption you hold that is stopping you from moving forward or doing something? What is the reason behind it?

Try using the steps in the previous exercise to work through your assumption and come to a different conclusion. Commit to acting based on the information you know or asking questions to gather more information.

# Identify Your Core Beliefs

Core beliefs are those beliefs you hold firmly. They indicate how you see yourself and others and how you view the world. They are usually rigid and inflexible and are formed in childhood or because of significant life events. Negative core beliefs are often related to the following:

- I am not good enough.
- I am unlovable.
- I am a terrible person.
- I am stupid.
- I am a defective human being.
- I am powerless.
- I am not safe.

Taking the time to analyze what you are thinking helps identify negative thinking. However, core beliefs are harder to identify because they hide below layers of problematic thoughts. You sometimes need to dig deep to find the underlying core belief. Uncovering your core beliefs might go something like this:

You didn't get a promotion at work after taking the initiative and staying late to finish projects. Your thoughts might be…

- I didn't get the promotion.
- I don't try hard enough.
- I can't do anything right.
- Because of this, I will never get promoted.
- The underlying core belief: I am not good enough.

You might have noticed the problematic thinking patterns in this thought process:

- Always and never—"I will never get promoted." These types of statements can leave you feeling hopeless.
- Fortune telling—"I will never get promoted." Never is a long time, and there is a good chance you will not always be in the same position.
- Ignoring the positive—"I can't do anything right." Throughout your life, there are probably many things you have done right.

You might have tried to combat these statements. You might think that you need to work harder or be a perfectionist. However, until you address the negative core belief that you are not good enough, your life could remain in a negative cycle.

If you tend to use one or more problematic thinking processes, you can create coping statements to counter the unhelpful thought patterns.

A coping statement is a statement that counters your most painful struggles and gets you to focus on where you have control or how you are feeling.

Coping Statements:

- **Degeneralize:** "Work is just one part of my life. It does not mean I am a failure. Not getting this promotion does not reflect on who I am."
- **Avoid assumptions:** "There is no evidence that I will never get a promotion. If I talk to my boss about where I can improve, I might get the next promotion."
- **Deal with core beliefs:** "I am good enough. I have this job and a good life. One promotion does not mean I am a failure."

Look over the different problematic thinking processes in Chapter 2. Now that you have spent more time paying attention to your thoughts, do you have a dominant style? Create coping statements to help you reframe your thoughts.

You might not completely believe your core beliefs, but even those you partially believe affect your behavior. For example, when going on a job interview, you tell yourself, "This is going to be a good interview." Despite not knowing the outcome, you dress appropriately, are well-groomed, have your resumé with you, and act professionally. You don't need to believe your statement to make good decisions.

Use coping statements to help deal with situations that repeat. For example, you consistently worry without proof that your boss is angry at you. Your coping message might be, "Everyone is in a bad mood sometimes. My boss's mood isn't about me." Whenever you notice you are personalizing the situation at work, repeat your coping statement.

# Your Turn: Rating Core Beliefs

When challenging core beliefs, think about how much you believe something. For example, you go out after work with some colleagues and forget to let your partner know you will be late. When you get home, she is angry that you did not call.

*Core belief:* I am always inconsiderate and not a good person.

*Ask yourself:* How often does my partner think I am inconsiderate? Does my partner think I am a terrible person? Rate your answers on a scale of 1–100 percent. You might decide your partner feels you are inconsiderate 20 percent of the time, meaning that you are considerate 80 percent of the time. Before believing this assumption, ask your partner if it is true. You might be surprised and find she only thinks you are inconsiderate occasionally and that 95 percent of the time, you are considerate.

*Your coping statement:* "Most of the time, I am considerate of my partner. Being inconsiderate occasionally does not make me a bad person. It does not define who I am. I am still a good person."

## Develop New Core Beliefs

Just as you challenged negative thinking processes and assumptions, you can test core beliefs by gathering evidence to prove or disprove the statement. Using the example that you did not get a promotion at work and that you believe, "I am not good enough," create a list of evidence to disprove your theory. Your list might include...

- I received promotions at my previous job.
- I recently got a raise at this company.
- My boss has complimented my work.
- I was asked to complete special projects.

These past experiences reflect that you are good enough. You are probably missing relevant information on why you didn't get the promotion. Rather than believing false, negative statements about yourself, ask your boss why and what you can do in the future to improve your work.

In Chapter 10, we discuss behavioral experiments, which test your predictions and core beliefs. For now, create a simple hypothesis about your belief and then gather evidence to prove or disprove your theories about yourself.

Write down a core belief you have about yourself. List any past experiences that go against this belief. Although you might not completely disprove the view, you might need to revise it because it is not always true. In the previous example, the core belief was changed from "I am always inconsiderate," to "I am inconsiderate on occasion." Base your core beliefs on who you are as a whole person, not what you did one time.

In this chapter, we discussed automatic thoughts, assumptions, and core beliefs. Automatic thoughts are those that pop into your head without consent and reflect how you view yourself, others, and the world around you. You can listen and change your automatic thoughts to change how you perceive and react to a situation. You typically base assumptions on incomplete information. Stopping to gather more details helps when making decisions. Core beliefs are deep-rooted beliefs about yourself that you can challenge in the same way you challenge thoughts.

# CHAPTER 4
# Understanding and Measuring Your Emotions

When you experience surges of emotion, your brain and body respond. For example, you have an important test coming up and whenever you think about it, you feel nervous. Your brain feels overwhelmed. You find it difficult to concentrate, and you are easily distracted. Your body feels tense, your breathing is a little faster than usual, and your hands become clammy. These emotions connect thoughts to behaviors.

In this chapter, we'll explore a variety of emotions and how they manifest in thoughts behaviors. We'll introduce methods to help you become more aware of your emotions and techniques for managing your feelings when they become overwhelming.

## Naming Your Emotions

How are you feeling today? Are you angry? Annoyed? Anxious? Happy? Embarrassed? Sad? Do you have mixed feelings? Although it is sometimes hard to identify what you feel, understanding your feelings helps manage reactions to them. Extreme emotions can be harmful to your health and cause you to react in negative ways. Studies have found intense negative emotions are linked to an increased risk of cardiovascular disease, immune system deficiencies, high blood pressure, and chronic pain. When you don't understand and manage emotions, your health, self-image, and relationships suffer.

Learning to identify both the emotion and its intensity provides a road map to managing the negative thought process behind the feeling. You can use your ABCD process to evaluate the negative thoughts for errors and challenge irrational points of view. Then you can change the unhelpful thoughts and, in turn, change your emotional state.

# Helpful vs. Unhelpful Emotions

All negative emotions are not bad. For example, sadness is considered a negative emotion, but when someone close to you dies, it is natural to feel sad. It signals, "I am experiencing a loss." However, when that sadness leads to depression, it becomes unhelpful and signals that you are having difficulty coping with the loss.

Unhelpful negative emotions usually indicate you believe you are not able to cope with the problem at hand. You view something in your situation as a threat to your safety or security. When you are experiencing these types of emotions, you usually lack compassion for yourself or others.

We often use alternate words to express our feelings. These terms might relate to the intensity of the basic emotion, be an expression or style of speaking, or could be a way of more accurately describing how you experience the basic feeling. For example, if you are feeling "nervous" about a job interview, you might not necessarily associate this with feeling scared or that you are in danger. A better description for you might be "I feel jittery" or "I have some concerns." Finding the right term also helps others understand you and build empathy.

Managing your emotions includes the following:

- Determining how you are feeling.
- Measuring the intensity of the feeling and describing it accurately.
- Deciding if the feeling is helpful or unhelpful.

Your thoughts, actions, and physical sensations all give you clues. Look over the following descriptions of emotions. Note the differences between healthy and unhealthy forms of feelings, the physical sensations you might feel, and alternate words used to describe the emotion to help you narrow down your emotion and determine if it is helpful or unhelpful.

## Nervousness vs. Anxiety

Nervousness and anxiety are both related to a sense of not being in control. You could feel powerless.

*Nervousness (healthy):* A situation in the present or the future threatens your sense of safety or security. You feel vulnerable. Low and moderate feelings of nervousness often activate a need to get something done.

*Anxiety or Panic (unhealthy):* Anxiety or panic is a less-healthy counterpart to nervousness. You perceive you cannot cope with the threat. Your fight-or-flight response is triggered, which is a physiological reaction to stress that increases heart rate, blood pressure, and glucose levels. Adrenalin levels go up, preparing you to either fight the threat or flee the situation.

*Alternate words:* worry, concern, apprehension, fear, agitation, tense, edgy, jitters, panic, uncertainty

*Physical sensations:* rapid heartbeat, shaking, sweating, stomachache, anxiety, dizziness

## Irritation and Frustration vs. Anger and Rage

These emotions are based on a sense of unfairness. You feel something must be changed.

*Irritation and frustration (healthy):* An obstacle is standing in the way of your perception of fairness and righteousness. It could be something that occurred in your past, is now occurring, or you fear will happen in the future. The larger you perceive the obstacle to be, the higher your level of frustration.

Frustration can be healthy because it signals that something is wrong and needs to be solved. It prevents you from ignoring an issue until it builds and you explode with anger or ignore it, allowing anger and resentment to simmer inside.

*Anger and rage (unhealthy):* Anger is the toxic manifestation of frustration. When you are angry, you don't believe you can handle the obstacle. Anger can lead to rage and hostility.

*Alternate words:* annoyed, irritated, bad-tempered, enraged, fuming, furious, hostile, livid, miffed, testy, touchy, displeased, cross, outrage, in a huff, hissy fit, mad

*Physical sensations:* grinding your teeth, clenching your fists, flushing, numbness, sweating, muscle tension

## Sadness vs. Depression

Sadness and depression are passive emotions and are a reaction to a sense of loss.

*Sadness (healthy):* A feeling based on the loss of something valuable and vital. Feelings of sadness are temporary. You know you will eventually feel better.

*Reactionary depression (unhealthy):* A harmful form of sadness that occurs after a loss that signals "I cannot cope with this loss." When you are depressed, you stop trying to improve your life situation. You feel a sense of hopelessness. Depression prevents you from accepting and mourning the loss and dealing with problems.

Reactionary depression is different from biological forms of depression. With biological depression, you have a chemical imbalance that causes you to feel depressed and think of the world as a painful place. In reactionary forms of depression, you react to an incident that colors your judgment.

*Major depression (unhealthy):* A medical condition that affects thoughts, feelings, behavior, and physical health. Depression is a lifelong condition that is much more than a temporary sadness. While some people have only one episode of depression, for many, it recurs throughout their lives.

Major depression can be a misleading term, as there isn't a "minor" depression. The term major is used to differentiate it from reactionary depression and to distinguish it as a medical condition rather than a general feeling of sadness.

*Alternate words:* disappointed, hurt, blue, distraught, down, heartbroken, melancholy, sorrowful, deflated, dejected, discouraged, dismayed, let down, grief, lonely, hopelessness, misery, dejection, despondency, gloomy, mopey, in a funk, dismal

*Physical sensations:* fatigue, crying, body aches and pains, stomachache, headache, changes in appetite

## Embarrassment vs. Guilt and Shame

When you feel embarrassment, guilt, or shame, you believe you have not lived up to self-imposed expectations.

*Embarrassment (healthy):* You feel somewhat responsible for something that has gone wrong. You assume others are judging you and your actions.

*Guilt and shame (unhealthy):* These are more extreme and toxic versions of embarrassment. You believe you should have control over the situation, and you are entirely responsible for the bad outcome. You do not think others will have empathy for your situation.

*Alternate words:* humiliated, degraded, discredited, disgraced, dishonored, self-conscious, uncomfortable, condemned, culpable, at fault, inexcusable, reprehensible, unforgivable, remorse, sorry, abashed, contrite, mortified, self-disgust

*Physical sensations:* blushing, feeling uncomfortable in social situations, insomnia, upset stomach, inability to look someone in the eye

## Disgust vs. Contempt

Disgust and contempt are forceful emotions that are similar to anger and rage. They result from disapproval of something you find unpleasant or offensive.

*Disgust (healthy):* A feeling of revulsion, aversion, or distaste to something that might cause you to withdraw from the object or person.

*Contempt (unhealthy):* A less-healthy form of disgust. You believe you are morally superior to another person; you think that the person is unworthy of your consideration.

*Alternate words:* revulsion, dislike, distaste, hatred, abhorrence, objection, loathing, disregard, scorn, aversion

*Physical sensations:* withdrawal from the object or person; nausea; facial expressions that include narrowing eyebrows, curled upper lip, and wrinkling nose

## Stress vs. Shock and Feeling Overwhelmed

Stress, shock, and feeling overwhelmed are all connected to agitation, either from an external event or from an internal struggle.

*Stress (healthy):* Emotional or mental strain when faced with demanding circumstances. The more things you need to deal with, the more stressed you are likely to feel. High levels of stress can lead to feeling overwhelmed and can develop from both good and bad experiences.

*Shock and feeling overwhelmed (unhealthy):* More intense and harmful versions of stress. These signal you are exhausted and exasperated; you are ready to shut down rather than continue to function.

*Alternate words:* distress, exasperation, frantic, unease, dismay, dread, strain, tension

*Physical sensations:* The fight-or flight-response is triggered, causing rapid heartbeat and an increase in adrenalin. When you feel overwhelmed, symptoms increase and can include chest pain, nausea, and dizziness.

## Envy vs. Jealousy

Both envy and jealousy involve believing you deserve something.

*Envy (healthy):* You want something that someone else has, although you don't necessarily want the other person not to have it, and you might be motivated to obtain this thing or something similar for yourself.

*Jealousy (unhealthy):* The fear that someone else will take something (or someone) you perceive as yours. It is the fear of losing something.

*Alternate words:* covet, green-eyed monster, resentment, rivalry, lusting

*Physical sensations:* feelings of unhappiness, tightening of jaw and mouth, pain in the pit of the stomach. Feelings of jealousy can include those of anxiety, such as racing heart. You might also feel a lump in your throat and breathlessness.

# Your Turn: Discover Underlying Attitudes

*The form accompanying this exercise is in Appendix C.*

Over the next three days, write down four events of the day. For example, going to work, cooking dinner, calling your mother, interacting with friends or coworkers, studying for an exam, or going on a trip.

Complete this exercise as soon after the event as possible. If you don't have time, complete it at the end of the day, visualizing what happened and replaying the details of the event in your mind. Think about and feel the emotion that you felt as the situation occurred. Imagine how your body felt and what you were thinking for clues to help the process.

Next to each event, write your emotion, using the descriptive words in the list of emotions to guide you. Rate the emotion's intensity on a scale of 1 to 10, with 10 being the most intense and 1 being the least. After three days, go back to see if there are one or two emotions you are experiencing more often than others.

You might be surprised at the results. For example, you don't think of yourself as an angry person, but after looking over your list, you realize that nearly half of the emotions you felt were related to anger or frustration. While this doesn't mean you are an angry person or that you spend most of your day feeling angry, evidence shows your underlying attitude is to feel anger when things don't go your way. You can create coping mechanisms and statements to reduce feelings of anger.

If you are having difficulty completing this exercise, try tracking your emotions the opposite way. Write down the main categories:

- Anxiety/Nervousness
- Anger
- Sadness/Depression
- Embarrassment/Guilt
- Disgust/Contempt
- Stress
- Envy/Jealousy

Each time you notice an emotion over the next several days, write down a brief description of the situation and a word that best describes how you are feeling. Rate each emotion on a scale of 1 to 10. As you continue, you might notice that you are experiencing certain emotions more than others.

Rating emotions helps determine which areas are most problematic. Sometimes, it is not the area you initially thought needed the most work. For example, you could begin CBT wanting to work on anger. After tracking your emotions and giving each a rating, you find that you experience sadness more often, and this becomes your primary issue. As you change your thinking process behind your dismay, the anger issues might disappear as well.

If you rate your emotions higher than a five, you could benefit from lowering the intensity first. If so, complete an ABCD worksheet to challenge your perspective and come up with coping thoughts. If you still can't calm down, try talking to a close friend, relative, or therapist.

## Mixed Emotions

Emotions are not always straightforward. Sometimes, you have mixed feelings, which are two competing sets of thoughts and emotions about the same situation. Let's say you have been dating someone for a few months. The two of you get along well and have fun together, you each want different things out of the relationship. While you want to get married, the other person is looking for a more casual relationship. After spending time together, you feel attached, accepted, and perhaps loved, but at the same time, you feel rejected, sad, and frustrated that this person does not want the same things. You end the relationship, knowing it's the best thing for you in the long run. However, you still feel upset and lonely. You miss spending time with a person who had become important to you. In this situation, you have mixed emotions: sadness and love.

Behind the emotions, you also have mixed thoughts. You might be thinking…

- The relationship will never be what I want it to be, but I miss him.
- There is someone else I find attractive, but I still want to be with my ex.

These mixed thoughts are often confusing, but they are not unhealthy.

An unhealthy reaction would be to intertwine thoughts and emotions. For example, you might think…

- This person doesn't care about me. (overgeneralization, mind reading)
- This person is an uncaring jerk. (personalization)
- This is evidence that I will never get married. (overgeneralization)
- Things will never work out for me. (black-and-white thinking)

The next time you feel mixed up and confused about a problem, stop and write all the emotions you feel and the thoughts connected to each one. Use your list to reflect on the feelings and gain a reasonable perspective that encourages acceptance and allows you to move on.

When dealing with an array of negative emotions, take a few minutes to bring yourself back to the present moment. Many negative emotions deal with the past or the future. Dealing with the present moment makes managing your mixture of emotions easier.

## Managing Feelings about Feelings

Sometimes, you have feelings about feelings, called *meta-emotions*. For example, you are angry at your child for breaking curfew. At the same time, you feel guilty for being mad because you believe you should be more understanding. Guilt is a secondary, or meta, feeling. At times, the secondary emotion becomes so strong it masks the original emotion and makes it more challenging to sort out your feelings and prevents you from actively dealing with the primary, or first, emotion.

Meta-emotions are a "double whammy." Not only do you put off dealing with the primary emotion, you now have a second emotion to manage.

Some people grew up believing emotions should remain hidden or that large displays of emotion were wrong. If this is the case, when you have strong feelings, you tell yourself it is wrong and try to squelch the emotion. When naming and evaluating your feelings, try to identify and deal with meta-emotions first.

## Your Turn: Create an Emotion Contract

Write down three situations when you felt emotional. Write down the emotion you felt and rate each one on a scale of 0 to 100. Include any actions you wanted to take because of your feelings. For example:

**Situation 1:** My spouse forgot to make the mortgage payment. Anger (70/100). I want to yell.

**Situation 2:** My friend called to tell me he can't go on vacation with me. He has done this in the past. Annoyance (50/100). I don't want to talk to him right now.

Does the incident or situation match your level of emotion? Does the intensity of your feeling signal an overreaction? If so, you might need to challenge the negative thought processes behind your emotions.

Create an emotion contract that states for the next week, you will not give in to feelings without thinking about the thoughts behind them. You will keep a thought log and complete an ABCD chart before letting the emotion fester. Sign and date your contract.

As you complete your ABCD log, come up with a new and healthier way of coping. Using the previous examples, you might come up with the following:

**Situation 1:** Frustration (40/100). Maybe my spouse is feeling overwhelmed right now. Instead of yelling at him, I could ask what is upsetting him and work together on a solution.

**Situation 2:** Stress and annoyance (30/100). I need to plan another trip or find someone else to go. In the future, I won't plan activities that rely on my friend.

## The Emotional Process

Your emotions affect you in many ways. The emotional process involves cognitive, physical, and behavioral reactions. When you understand how these reactions interact, it is easier to break the cycle.

You can make changes anywhere in the cycle to create positive change. For example, if you are dealing with sadness and mild depression, you could have the following reactions:

*Cognitive:* You have difficulty focusing or paying attention.

*Physical:* You have difficulty sleeping or sleep too much.

*Behavioral:* You avoid going out with friends or stay in bed all day.

Suppose you wake up thinking, "My life isn't any good. I don't even want to get out of bed today." Staying in bed will probably make you feel worse. You lie in bed, thinking about all the reasons you shouldn't get up and go to work. You ruminate about everything bad in your life. Later, you feel guilty for not going to work. By the end of the day, your depression has deepened.

Now, suppose that you wake up thinking, "My life isn't any good. I don't even want to get out of bed today, but I know it is best to get up and get moving." And so you do. You get up, you shower, get dressed, have breakfast, and force yourself to go to work. Once there, you start to feel better. By changing your behavior, you changed your emotional state. You broke the cycle by changing one reaction. Once you did that, it became much easier to change your thoughts and look at the positive in your life.

## Cognitive Reactions

In Chapter 2, you learned about the different problematic thinking processes. When you experience an unhelpful emotional reaction, you might be using one of these thinking processes:

- *Black-and-white thinking* commonly leads to depression and anger.
- *Personalization* commonly leads to guilt and anxiety.
- *Overgeneralizing* might lead to depression and anger.
- *Ignoring the positive* can lead to stress and worry.
- *Mind reading* can lead to anxiety and embarrassment.
- *Catastrophizing and fortune-telling* lead to anxiety, worry, and depression.

# Physical Reactions

Emotions don't just live in your mind. Research shows they show up in your body, too. For example, when you feel nervous, you feel "butterflies in your stomach." The basic emotions—anger, fear, disgust, happiness, sadness, and surprise—are associated with bodily sensations and reactions in the upper chest, such as heart rate and breathing. Other physical manifestations of emotions include specific facial expressions and changes in the brain triggered by emotional reactions.

More complex emotions include anxiety, love, depression, contempt, pride, and shame. These are often felt more deeply in the body. The sensations include regions such as the legs, hands, heart, and head.

Review the list of emotions and the corresponding physical sensations at the start of the chapter and take note of the ones you feel regularly. Pay attention to your physical reactions and sensations to help determine whether your responses and associated thought processes are helpful or unhelpful. When you experience helpful and healthy emotions, the associated physical responses help you react swiftly to dangers and take advantage of opportunities. Consider the following scenarios:

**Scenario 1:** You're walking along a city street alone in an unfamiliar area, and your directions take you down an alley. Your muscles tense, your heartbeat speeds up, your body is on high alert. It is your body's way of telling you to be careful.

**Scenario 2:** You prepare to give a presentation at work. You feel nervous, your mind feels more focused, and your adrenaline helps you get ready for the presentation and remain steady during the talk.

While mild physical sensations from emotions can be helpful, more pronounced physical feelings might interfere with healthy behaviors and reactions. Think back to giving a presentation at work. Instead of feeling mildly nervous, you feel very anxious. Your heart is beating rapidly, and your breathing becomes fast and shallow. You feel tightness in your chest, shakiness in your hands, and pins and needles in your legs. The more intense your physical reaction, the more you tell yourself the presentation is going to be terrible, and the more you want to avoid it. In a nutshell, the emotions and physical sensations are too intense. Rather than helping you take advantage of the opportunity, they end up contributing to your failure.

By paying attention to physical sensations in your body, you can better connect to your emotions and thoughts. For example, if you pay attention to the butterflies in your stomach as soon as they happen, you recognize that you're nervous and accept it. Instead of giving in to negative thoughts and uncomfortable body sensations, you can use the ABC technique to challenge your thinking.

# Behavioral Reactions

Your behavior provides clues to whether your feeling and thinking are helpful or unhelpful. In general, useful behaviors are those that are constructive; unhelpful behaviors are those that are self-destructive. Obvious self-destructive behaviors include substance abuse and self-harming behaviors, but there are other nonhelpful behaviors, too. These include the following:

- Telling someone off or confronting someone without learning the facts of a situation.
- Avoiding or escaping a situation, such as running out of a meeting or not getting on a plane.
- Not doing anything—not taking care of hygiene, not doing pleasurable things, and withholding self-rewards.

Instead of giving in to these behaviors, use your emotion contract, and add a new, positive action to perform over the next month. For example:

- Before you confront someone, you will go for a 10-minute walk. Then ask for information and start a discussion rather than jumping to conclusions and reacting angrily.
- If you anticipate a stressful situation, you will give yourself 20 minutes to relax and prepare.
- Instead of giving in to depression, you will create a schedule that includes the activities you enjoy.

Changing your behavior, even slightly, changes your perspective and reduces negative emotions.

# Learned Emotions

Emotions are sometimes triggered through associations and learned reactions known as conditioning. For example, suppose when you were in school, you took exams in a blue room. During the exams, you felt anxious. Perhaps you had a negative experience, such as failing an oral exam in front of your classmates. Now, as an adult, whenever you sit in a blue room, you automatically feel a change in your heart rate, breathing, and muscle tension. Initially, you might connect this with being scared, but the longer you remain in the situation, the more your emotions build. You have fearful thoughts and a strong desire to get out of the room as soon as possible. The longer you stay, the more noticeable your reaction. You might or might not be aware that your response has anything to do with the room being blue.

Conditioning occurs when your brain and body learn to associate an emotion with a set of situations or stimuli. The body sensations become connected to the stimuli, which then triggers the feeling.

Because you might not remember or be aware of the association between your feelings and certain situations, it is sometimes hard to know if it is a learned emotion. Some fears that frequently result from conditioning include…

- Phobias such claustrophobia, travel anxiety, heights, needles.
- Social anxiety.
- Depression associated with traumas.
- Public speaking.

If you are experiencing feelings because of conditioning, this statement might apply to you: "I often feel this way when I'm in this type of setting. I know I'm not in danger, but I cannot help but feel this way." To determine if your emotions are associated with past experiences, complete the emotion chart from the previous exercises. Write down the date, time, and what you felt. Add facts about your situation, such as where you are, what you are doing, and who is with you. These variables help you find commonalities to give you clues about past experiences.

You might write down the following:

Monday, December 16, 2019. Conference room meeting. I felt very nervous, my hands were shaking, and I had an urge to escape. I was sensitive to any critique of my work. Ten people were present; one person in charge who was doing the most talking. The chairs were comfortable; there were windows in the room and blue paint on the walls.

Once you write down the details, ask yourself…

1. What did I think once the emotion started?
2. Are these thoughts relevant here?
3. Are there negative thoughts about the present situation I can challenge?

Your answers to these questions might give you clues to where your nervousness and fear originated. For example, you might have answered:

1. "When I am in the conference room, I think my boss is going to yell at me and give me a bad report. I don't want to ask any questions or offer any advice."
2. "I know this is not really going to happen and that I am reacting emotionally because I feel anxious. My boss has not yelled at me during a conference before, and I have no reason to think he is going to this time."
3. "I can calm down in conferences because I know that I have been asked to join the meeting. I am a valuable member of the team and have information to share."

You can now look back to see if there were similar situations in your past. What does this situation remind you of? "When I was in junior high, I remember that I took my exams in a small blue room. The teachers walked around the room, openly criticizing me and making me nervous. I remember feeling like I wanted to run away, and I sometimes skipped school when I needed to take a test in that room."

If you think you are dealing with a conditioned emotional response, one way to handle it is through exposure techniques. This method slowly introduces you to a fearful situation until you no longer feel nervous or anxious. It is covered in detail in Chapter 17.

Managing your emotions begins with identifying them and the thoughts behind them. Your body can give you clues to how you are feeling. Different emotions evoke different bodily sensations, such as butterflies in your stomach from nervousness. When you better understand what you are feeling and why, you can challenge negative thought processes. It is possible to experience more than one emotion at a time, called *mixed emotions*. For example, you can feel happy that you got a new job and nervous about your first day.

# PART 2

# CBT Techniques

CBT isn't just a single strategy; it is a combination of different techniques to help you think, feel, and act in helpful and constructive ways. In this part, you learn many of the methods you need to put CBT into practice in your daily life.

Imagery, relaxation techniques, meditation, and mindfulness all help you challenge, test, and change automatic thoughts and images that cause distress. The different exercises in this section help you practice the strategies, so you can use them in many different situations.

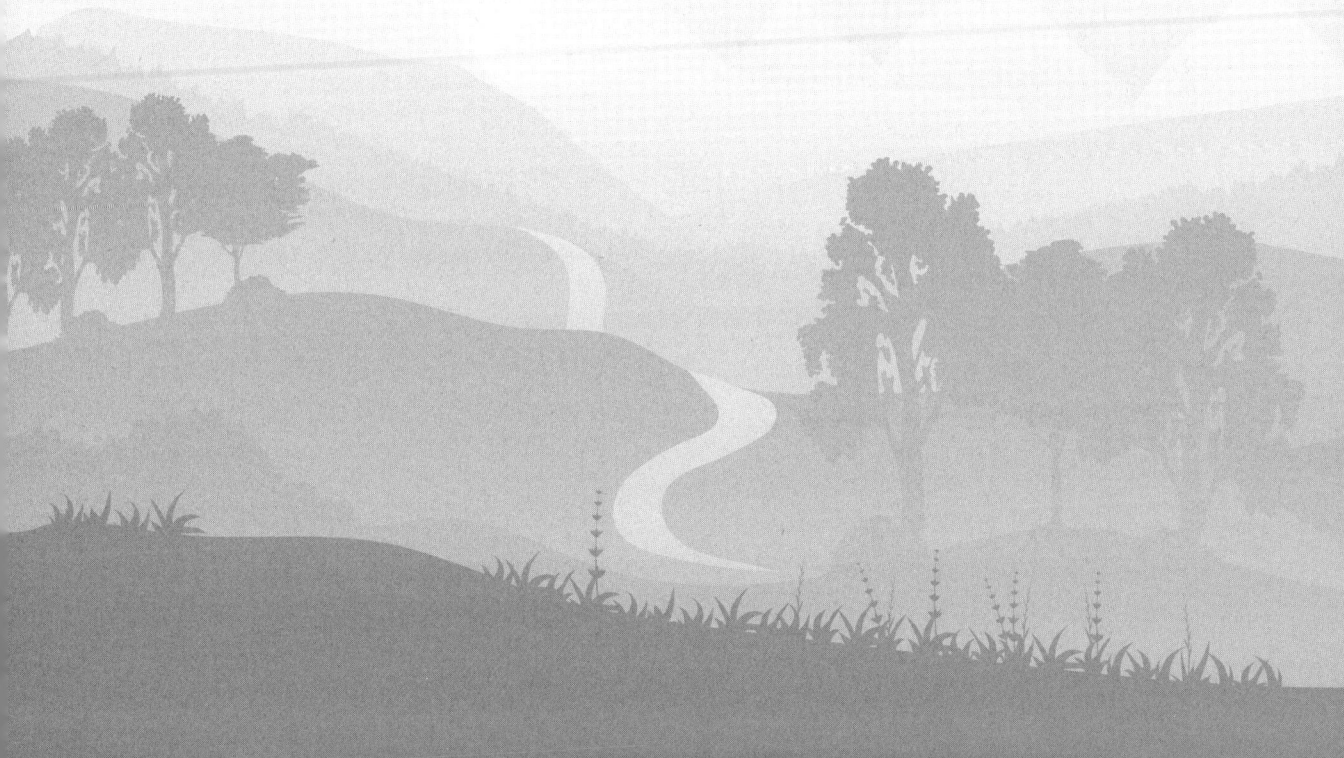

# CHAPTER 5
# Setting Goals for Getting Better

When you picked up this book, what did you have in mind? Did you know what you want to change? You might have depression, anxiety, or anger issues and want to work directly on those. You might have chronic pain or want to be more assertive. You might not be sure what is going on but you feel overwhelmed in your life.

Whatever brought you to this book, you are ready for change. You might not know where you want to end up, but you know you want to feel better. This chapter is about getting from where you are to feeling better. You'll learn how to set goals and how to develop a plan of action.

## Setting Goals

You need a goal before beginning work on improving specific areas of your life. Goals should be specific, measurable, and achievable. They should have a time limit, be positive, and be relevant to your life. Think about what you want to do, rather than what you want to stop doing.

### What Is a SMART Goal?

We use goals in every area of our life, sometimes without realizing it. "I need to go to the store after work and buy milk and bread" is a goal. Goals give us structure and accountability to work toward a better way of living. Without goals, you open yourself to chaos and lost opportunities. The acronym SMART helps ensure that your plan has essential components.

***S—Specific***—Your goal should be specific. Instead of "I want to have a healthy lifestyle," try "I will eat vegetables every day for the next two weeks."

***M—Measurable***—You need to know whether you have reached your goal or the milestones to indicate you are on your way. It's difficult to determine if you "have a healthy lifestyle," but it is easy to decide if you ate vegetables today.

***A—Attainable***—Can you achieve this goal? Consider the effort and time your plan requires. Is that something you can do? Is it reasonable to expect you to reach the goal? Setting unreachable goals sets you up for failure.

***R—Relevant***—Is your goal relevant to your life? Does the plan fit in with your values? While the goal of eating vegetables is standard, running a marathon next month when you don't run every day is not relevant to your life. Decide if this goal fits your life.

***T—Timely***—Do you have a start and finish line? "I will eat vegetables every day for two weeks" gives you an end. Two weeks from now, you can look back to determine if you met your goal. When goals go on for an indeterminate length of time, you lose motivation.

Let's walk through the process of determining and setting goals with an example. When you created your emotion log, you might have noticed you angered easily, or you react defensively whenever someone corrects you or gives you feedback you view as unfavorable. Your emotion log might look like this:

| A: Activating Event | B: Belief or Thoughts | C: Consequences or Responses to Change |
|---|---|---|
| My boss pointed out some mistakes in my work. | He never liked me anyway. He tries to find mistakes. | Became irritated. Snapped at coworkers even though I was mad at my boss. |
| My partner did not like my choice of restaurants for dinner. | My partner never pays attention to what I want. My partner is selfish. | I barely spoke to my partner during dinner. |

As you look over your chart, you notice whenever someone gives you feedback or disagrees, you view it as criticism and become angry or irritated. You want to change how you respond. Setting specific goals is vital to the process. Ask yourself…

- How do I want to feel during these encounters?
- How do I want to come across? Open or closed? Flexible or rigid?
- How would I prefer to behave during these encounters?

- If I'd had a different reaction, how would my view of the situation differ?
- If I did not get upset so quickly, what parts of my life would improve?

The next step is to decide how you want to feel and act. You might say:

> I want to feel confident that I can handle feedback from other people. I want to act pleasantly even when someone disagrees with me.

Using the list in Chapter 2, think about which problematic thought processes you use when you overreact. In this example, it is overgeneralization and ignoring the positive.

Now it is time to create a goal:

> When someone criticizes me or gives me feedback, I will first thank them for their feedback and later decide if their feedback is relevant.

You can also create a coping statement that you turn to whenever you begin to feel irritated because someone gives feedback. Your coping message might be:

> She is expressing her perspective; it is not a reflection of me as a person. I receive positive feedback regularly.

If you're have a difficult time creating a specific goal, imagine a situation where you displayed behavior you do not like, such as irritation and anger, at feedback. Consider several different endings to a scenario, using different reactions in each. Then choose the one you prefer—the ideal way you want to react to feedback. Try to put that image into words. How do you feel? What are your thoughts? How does the situation change? Does your behavior change? Does your mood change?

If you have trouble reaching goals, you could be choosing end results that are too general. Try making them more specific, or break down goals into small chunks and take one step at a time.

# Your Turn: Ladder Rungs

*The form accompanying this exercise is in Appendix C.*

When creating goals, it's easy to be too ambitious. You're eager to make changes in your life and to see the result. However, taking shortcuts and skipping steps makes it more difficult to meet your goal.

In the previous example, your goal was, "When someone criticizes me or gives me feedback, I will first thank them for their feedback and later decide if their feedback is relevant." This image is your end result.

Goals work best when you create a series of steps, with each stage moving you closer to the desired result. Think of these steps like rungs on a ladder. Think about past actions and list times you reacted poorly to others' feedback. What was your worst reaction? This is your starting point—the first rung on your ladder.

Continue to list more moderate behaviors, working your way toward your desired reaction. Each of these reactions becomes a rung on the ladder, and each becomes a goal. The ladder provides a way to monitor your progress and gives you a sense of accomplishment as you move up the rungs.

# Define Your Motivation

Change is never easy. It is comfortable to fall back into old habits, even if those habits are negative or unhealthy. Don't become discouraged. With focus, determination, and the right goals, you can achieve results.

Suppose you suffer from anxiety. Your anxiety level rises when you are in a crowd. You feel dizzy, nauseous, and shaky, so you avoid crowded spaces. You stay away from the city, don't eat in restaurants, and shop online exclusively to skip shopping at a mall.

So far, this strategy works; when you only go to selected activities, you avoid the unpleasant feeling of having a panic attack, but it also limits your life. You stay home while friends head to the city or dinner for a night out. You limit where you work to small companies with only a few employees. You have chosen to compromise your lifestyle to avoid having a panic attack.

Think about what your life would be like if you didn't worry about anxiety. Where would you go? What type of work would you do? Create an image of what you want — this is your end goal. This is the top rung of your ladder. It is also your motivation to change. The more you grow this image, the more you want to achieve it.

## Weighing the Pros and Cons

Without realizing it, you considered the costs and benefits of going to certain places and determined that the price (anxiety) is more than you are willing to pay, regardless of the benefit. To change your thoughts, you need to reevaluate the costs and benefits.

A cost-benefit analysis is a tool to weigh the pros and cons of making a change. It is sometimes helpful to complete two cost-benefit examinations—one for continuing your present behavior and one for changing. Using our previous example, the cost-benefit analysis for using CBT to overcome anxiety might look like this:

*Pros:*

- I will learn to go out in public without having a panic attack.
- I can try new restaurants.
- I can join my friends when they go to the city.
- I can look for a better-paying job.
- I can look for a job I like better.

*Cons:*

- I will have to face my anxiety.
- I will have to face my fears and start going out.
- It will be scary and uncomfortable.

You can use a cost-benefit analysis to show the benefits and disadvantages of most decisions. For significant ones, break them down into smaller decisions. For example, using the previous model, you might look at changing just one area, such as going out to dinner.

*Pros of going to dinner with friends:*

- I enjoy my friends' company.
- I can try new foods.

*Cons of going to dinner with friends (or reasons to avoid going out to dinner):*

- I don't need to worry about my anxiety.
- I can relax at home.
- I don't spend as much money.

Be sure to list every pro and con that comes to mind. The cost-benefit analysis allows you to see both sides of an argument. It enables you to make an informed and rational decision.

## Positive vs. Negative Motivation

There are two types of motivation: positive and negative. With positive motivation, you work toward something pleasurable. Negative motivation is doing something to avoid discomfort or pain.

Imagine two people with the same job: One goes to work because he doesn't want to get fired and risk losing his home. The second person goes to work because he feels a sense of pride, independence, and financial stability. The first is negatively motivated; the second is positively motivated.

Negative motivation works but rarely leaves you with a sense of satisfaction and well-being. Positive motivation provides an inner force—a reason to keep going. It is looking at what you want rather than what you don't want. Consider your reason for wanting to change; is it framed positively or negatively? Sometimes, it is a matter of changing the wording:

*Negative:* I wish to change because I don't want to be left behind when my friends go out.

*Positive:* I want to change because I enjoy spending time with my friends.

The results are the same: going out to dinner with friends. One involves avoiding a situation (being left behind); the other involves an enjoyable outcome (spending time with my friends.) Your goals, or rewards, can be tangible—a new car—or intangible—enjoyment, respect, or happiness. When creating goals, ask yourself, "What do I have to gain?" rather than, "What am I going to lose if I don't do this?"

## Making Sure the Goal Is Yours

Have you heard a college student say, "I am majoring in science because that's what my parents want." The goal is "I am going to college and will graduate with a degree in science." But it isn't the student's goal; it is her parents' goal. Before committing to a plan, make sure you are the one who wants the result.

Suppose your goal is to have a cleaner house. You decided on this goal because you visited your brother and sister-in-law, and their home was spotless. When you came home, you looked around and decided your house didn't measure up. You now want a cleaner home. But do you want that because you want it, or do you want a cleaner home because you think you should want it? We work harder to accomplish goals when the result is something we want.

Listing the benefits of your goal can help. Focus on what you will get when you reach the goal. For example, if your goal is to lose 15 pounds, the benefits include a lower risk of diabetes, improved overall health, increased sense of well-being, and more energy. These benefits directly affect you. If one of your reasons is "My spouse thinks I should lose weight," your goal is for your spouse, not yourself. Look at your benefits and determine if your goal is yours or someone else's.

## Your Turn: Create a Cost-Benefit Analysis

*The form accompanying this exercise is in Appendix C.*

Create your cost-benefit analysis on a current problem you have. Use two columns labeled "Costs/Disadvantages" and "Benefits/Advantages." Write down every cost and benefit you think of, no matter how small. Weigh them against one another to see which option brings the most benefit.

Continue with the cost-benefit, using short-term and long-term pros and cons. Be sure to write the pros as a positive rather than as avoiding a negative. Use this tool to determine your risk and how both changing and staying the same affects your life. Use the positives to stay motivated.

## Your Turn: Create Coping Flash Cards

In a previous exercise, you created a ladder with steps to reach your goal. You should focus on one rung of the ladder at a time and continue moving forward until you achieve the desired behavior. As you start working on each level, create coping flash cards. These are small cards, such as index cards, to carry with you as a reminder of a positive statement to help when you are in a stressful situation.

First, list negative thoughts that could interfere with completing the goal. Each negative thought should have an index card. Turn the card over and write the opposite—a positive and realistic view to replace the negative thinking.

When you notice yourself thinking (or saying) the negative thought, pull out the corresponding card and read the positive alternative you wrote down. Try reading it aloud and repeating it several times.

## Maintaining Your Progress

It's essential to commit to reaching a goal. It is just as vital to maintain progress. Your commitment is a promise to yourself to make positive changes in your life and to continue using the skills you learn in this book to maintain those changes.

Following are the three levels of commitment:

- *Mental commitment:* A promise you make to yourself when you first decide to make a change. Mental commitments alone are easy to break.
- *Commitment made in writing:* A higher level of commitment. When you write a commitment down, you are more likely to keep the promise.
- *Commitment made by telling others:* When you share your goal with at least one other person, you strengthen your resolve to keep your commitment. Look for people who can provide positive support and encouragement.

If you are not comfortable sharing your goals, at least write down your commitment and place it somewhere you will see it every day to help reinforce your purpose and motivation.

# Tips for Setting Goals

*Behavior or feelings?* You can create goals based on how you want to behave or how you want to feel. When creating goals about feelings, focus on having positive emotions such as happiness, hopefulness, and pride. If you currently experience strong negative emotions, aim toward a less-intense reaction, such as moving from rage to annoyance.

*What goal will make the most difference?* Consider what behaviors have the most negative effect on your life and which are most likely to impact other problem behaviors. If you change the first behavior in a chain of reactions, it can result in modifying several behaviors.

*Limit your goals to improving one behavior at a time.* You want to focus on one fundamental behavior, such as quitting smoking or losing 10 pounds, rather than monitoring several elements of your health at the same time. Once you accomplish one goal, move on to focus on a separate area.

*Think about broad goals,* such as family, relationships, or work. Write down three issues you want to work on and list the pros and cons of each.

*Cost-benefit analysis can be used in many areas of your life,* including behaviors, emotions, thoughts, beliefs, and problem solving. You can modify your analysis to look at short-term or long-term solutions. It works best if you write statements in pairs: What is the advantage of making a change? How would that translate to a disadvantage of not making the change?

You need goals when making changes in your life. They provide focus and an outline of what you want to achieve. SMART goals are specific, measurable, attainable, relevant, and timely. It is easier to work toward goals when you approach them from a positive point of view–that is, when you work on something you want to do rather than something you want to stop. The cost-benefit analysis looks at the pros and cons of a goal to help with decision making.

# CHAPTER 6
# Visualization and Imagery

Visualization and imagery are potent tools frequently used in CBT to create positive changes. Spontaneous images, much like automatic thoughts, can be a result of distorted thinking. In this chapter, you will learn how to use visualization when handling difficult situations, as well as find ways to control mental images.

## Using Visualization

You probably use visualization every day without even realizing it. It is the act of using your imagination to create mental pictures and images. It either occurs spontaneously, or you consciously develop images in your mind. For example, a coworker suggests you meet for drinks after work. You might automatically picture a scene of the two of you at the bar, holding a glass and chatting. The more you visualize the image, the more details you fill in. You put your perspective into the details and use this visualization in your decision making.

When creating the image, you use past experiences, your current mood, and your feelings about your coworker. If you don't know your coworker well, you might envision stilted conversation. If you have enjoyed past discussions, you might see the two of you laughing and talking. The more details you put in, the sharper the image in your mind becomes—and the more you believe the image.

The images in your mind can be positive or negative. When your coworker suggested meeting, you could have conjured an image of stilted conversation. You might have seen yourself trying to escape an awkward situation. In this case, you might have decided not to go.

Just as you can change your thoughts, you can change the images in your mind. You can choose and control the scene. Using the previous example, if your first image was negative, you could decide to change it. When replacing an image, try to incorporate all your senses. Take a deep breath and imagine what you would smell, the feel of the glass in your hand, and what you see. The more senses you bring to your image, the more immersed you become in the new situation. As you add details and imagine yourself having a good time, you might realize you are looking forward to getting to know your coworker.

Whenever you face an awkward situation, create a scene in your mind. Imagine the problem and imagine yourself dealing with the situation. Picture yourself feeling confident. How do you look? Are you standing up straight, a smile on your face? What are you wearing? Who is with you? Where are you? Imagine yourself combating and challenging your negative thoughts. Practicing CBT techniques through visualization makes it easier to use the strategies when you need them.

Some people find it helpful to imagine a television with the remote in their hand. When your visualization is a picture of an event that causes anxiety or distress, change the channel and create a different, more pleasurable scene. When you feel anxious, remember you can change the channel to view something else.

# Facing Emotional Images

There might be times when you have an image in your mind that provokes anxiety, anger, or sadness. You don't want to see it and try to distract yourself by thinking of something else. Not thinking about it makes you feel better—at least in the short term. Unfortunately, avoidance reinforces your fear of dealing with the image; it keeps you emotionally connected to the image and prevents you from gaining control over it and the situation it represents.

Many people who live with anxiety use avoidance to lessen their discomfort. Thinking about visualizing or imagining a situation that triggers anxiety often produces just as much fear as if you were physically there. Using visualization helps you learn strategies for coping with stressful events. Avoiding them deprives you of the opportunity to practice the skills.

Desensitization is a method of regularly facing a scene, either in real life or in your mind. Each time you go through it, the emotion decreases. Sometimes, it is necessary to imagine a situation many times until you no longer have an intense adverse reaction. When that happens, go through it again, this time employing CBT techniques to find ways to cope. Desensitization is a process frequently used to help individuals unlearn phobias and anxieties.

For example, suppose you have a fear of dogs. Closing your eyes and imagining coming face to face with a dog raises your anxiety level. You start shaking, and your heart rate increases. The more vividly you create the scene in your mind, the more your anxiety increases. You can use desensitization to lower your anxiety. To start, write down five images reflecting five levels of difficulty, beginning with the easiest level and progressing to the most difficult. In the example of overcoming a fear of dogs, your levels might look something like this:

*Level 1:* Imagine yourself in a room with a dog that is locked in a crate or small dog run.

*Level 2:* Picture the same scene, this time with the dog on a leash where it cannot reach you.

*Level 3:* Imagine the dog on a leash, but he can reach you.

*Level 4:* Imagine sitting in the room, petting the dog.

*Level 5:* Visualize the dog sitting on your lap or lying by your feet.

Each time you do the visualization exercise, commit to picturing the image for 10 minutes. Hold the image in your mind before allowing your thoughts to move to something else. Use the same picture until your fear subsides and the next image provokes moderate anxiety to keep you from moving too fast through the levels. This technique lowers the risk of becoming emotionally overwhelmed.

If you find any of the images too upsetting, revise it to lessen the intensity and save the more vivid picture for the next rung in your hierarchy. Add as many levels as you need to reach your goal.

# Reacting to Spontaneous Imagery

Automatic thoughts sometimes come as pictures and images in your mind, often from something that makes you feel unsettled, either from your past or in anticipation of the future. They can range from small upsetting situations to traumatic events. Flashbacks and nightmares are other forms of spontaneous emotions and thoughts. Because automatic or involuntary images are usually brief and fleeting, you might dismiss the picture as quickly as it appears and might not be conscious of the image you created.

Suppose you argue with your boss. At home that evening, images of the disagreement replay in your mind. You see your boss frowning and scowling. You imagine him firing you. By the next morning, you are so worried about losing your job, you don't want to go to work.

Instead of imagining your boss angry, suppose you think about your boss listening to your side of the disagreement. You remain calm and look forward to resolving the issue the next day. You have the power to change negative images, just as you do with automatic thoughts.

## Solving Problems

Everyone becomes overwhelmed with problems at some point. Visualization can help find solutions. For example, suppose your in-laws are coming for dinner. Your partner was called into work and expects to be there for several hours. That leaves you with the bulk of the preparations. There is a list of things that need to get done—shopping, cleaning, preparing the food. You can do it, but the plan was to work with your partner; now, you are overwhelmed. Your thoughts include, "I will never get this done by myself," or "Dinner is going to be a disaster." At dinnertime, everything is fine, but you are irritable and wish your in-laws would just go home.

Your automatic negative thought process throughout the day was "never going to get it done" and "it is going to be a disaster." The pictures in your mind reflected these thoughts. You went through the day believing these thoughts and images and even though the dinner did get done, you didn't enjoy it and just wanted it to be over.

Try changing the images to help you solve problems. Picture what you are going to do each time a problem comes up. How are you going to solve it? What are you going to do? Instead of picturing yourself frazzled, imagine yourself working through each step. For example, think about the most concerning issue and the steps to resolve it. Maybe you are worried because the menu you created with your partner is too time consuming, especially when you need to complete the other tasks. Imagine the dinner if you changed the meal. Can you picture it working then?

## Testing Your Image

Sometimes, you base images on your imagination, not reality. For example, if you are an experienced cook, imagining a burnt dinner is not realistic. Likewise, if your in-laws have always been kind and understanding, imagining them as judgmental is not realistic. Test images to find out if there is any evidence to back up the image. You might ask yourself…

- Have I ever thrown a dinner party before that ended in a total disaster?
- Have my in-laws ever treated me disrespectfully?

Once you look at the situation more realistically, you determine that your images don't fit. You change the images to match what is happening.

## Changing the Image

Distressing images are usually exaggerated and not based on the reality of the situation. Take a step back to examine the pictures you created and decide how you can change them to reflect what is going on around you more closely.

Thoughts frequently come in a combination of words and pictures. The most highly charged memories often occur in the form of images. When you remember the event, you also recognize and experience the emotions again. Image rescripting is a way of changing a painful memory to one with a positive and empowering ending. This type of process breaks the negative emotional connection to the previous event.

There are three steps to the process of rescripting:

*Step 1:* Relive the event and the accompanying emotions.

*Step 2:* Create a different ending. Don't change the event itself, but extend the image to include your new conclusion. For example, your parents harshly criticized you when you were young. Now as an adult, you still feel shame when you think back to those times. Visualize one such event, but don't stop at the criticism; instead, add to the image and picture yourself leaving home and moving to a safe environment. If this has not happened yet, visualize yourself in the future when you are secure in your home.

*Step 3:* Nurture yourself, but yourself at the age of the traumatic event. For example, if you suffered an abusive event when you were eight years old, you would nurture the eight-year-old child. To do this, ask yourself what words of reassurance could have helped you. What information would have made you feel better at the time? For example, "I know one day, I will grow up and have a loving family and a happy home. I am a lovable person. The way my parents treat me is not a reflection of my worth."

Twice a day for a week, imagine the extended ending and nurture yourself. Once you complete the three steps as well as the daily practice sessions, the negative emotions should start to lessen.

The first step of image rescripting is often emotionally painful. It is recommended you work with a therapist or a trusted relative or friend when completing this process if you are trying to change a particularly traumatic or painful memory.

## Changing the Focus

Rather than changing the entire image, you can choose to change the direction of the picture. When you are upset, you usually see the situation from only one perspective. For example, when imagining the first day of a new job, you probably see either yourself or the faces of others. You might see yourself standing awkwardly and appearing lost, or you might mostly visualize your new coworkers staring at you. You see things in one direction.

This strategy involves changing your image to look at it from both sides, making both models positive. Using the image of your first day at a job, imagine your coworkers receptive and smiling, and you are walking over to introduce yourself.

## Completing the Story

As with automatic thoughts, when you are upset, angry, sad, or anxious, you might stop your image at the worst moment. For example, suppose you want to post a selfie on Instagram, but you are worried that nobody cares or nobody wants to see what you are doing. You worry that nobody will like your picture, which you see as a validation of your social standing. You have posting anxiety, which prevents you from maintaining connections on social media. You imagine posting the picture and repeatedly checking. No one liked it. Then you stop the image because it is painful for you to think no one bothered to pay attention. You carry this image with you for the rest of the day, feeling rejected and insecure.

Spontaneous images are often fleeting. They flash before your eyes and then are gone. When these images are negative, they can leave you feeling sad, angry, or depressed—whichever emotion you relate to the scene. However, you can make a conscious effort to finish the image—to complete the story and give it a happy ending.

Imagine that you return to Instagram later and your picture has garnered likes. Once you complete the story, you don't feel as bad. Instead of your insecurities affecting your entire day, you focus on the complete story, making it a positive experience.

## Your Turn: Create Your Imagery

You can use imagery to prepare yourself for an upcoming stressful situation and desensitize yourself to cope better. For example, suppose your employer has laid off some of your coworkers. You expect additional layoffs. You know there is a chance you are next. Visualize the scene when you find out you are out of a job. Repeat the image until you feel less emotional about it. If you do this for several days, when it does happen, you are better able to cope.

Practice by thinking about an upcoming situation causing you concern. It could relate to your job, your personal life, or a relationship. Create an image of the scene with as much detail as possible. Recall this image several times a day to help you let go of the intense emotion surrounding it to help you approach the situation calmly.

Even famous athletes use visualization. It not only improves performance but helps relieve fear and anxiety. Athletes such as Michael Jordan and Tiger Woods indicate visualization helps them perform their best.

## Create Coping Skills

Besides using visualization to cope with your current situations, you can use imagery to learn and practice coping skills. This strategy combines several different CBT techniques. As with all visualization techniques, start by creating an image of an action you plan to do. Then break down the scene to practice each part. This type of approach is useful for complex situations, such as job interviews or social interactions.

Using overly dramatic or exaggerated visualizations sometimes helps. Think of a play you have seen; the actors might have exaggerated certain lines to make a point, this uses the same concept. Be overly dramatic in your visualizations to emphasize certain behaviors or feelings. For example, you are incredibly nervous before a job interview. You want to give a good impression and convey you are capable, well-spoken, attentive, and curious. In this type of visualization, focus on each element individually. First, visualize the interview and concentrate on being well-spoken. Imagine yourself as extremely articulate and well beyond the level you need to achieve your goal.

Continue this visualization until you are comfortable with the image. Next, work on a different aspect of the interview, such as being attentive. In your visualization, pay attention to every word and gesture. Continue going through each element until you have visualized all the different parts. Lastly, combine them to create one overly dramatic visualization. This type of imaging helps you break down an overwhelming situation into small chunks. Sometimes you can practice each part separately; sometimes you can practice it in its entirety.

You can combine visualization with other CBT techniques. For example, if you feel nervous about getting a flu shot, you could use imaging with the deep breathing exercises described in Chapter 7. You might also use visualization when rewriting your self-talk, as explained in Chapter 9, or when revising perfectionistic behavior, as described in Chapter 12.

## Your Turn: Keynote-Behavior Visualizations

A keynote behavior is a defining behavior that changes the entire perception and experience of an incident in one primary action. It is an action that culminates in your feelings about a situation. For example, if you are afraid of riding the subway, you might find stepping on the subway train and having the doors close behind you the most frightening. This is your keynote behavior.

Visualization is useful in these types of situations because once you change that one behavior, you alter your perception, and further actions change as well. When using imaging to change a keynote behavior, repeatedly visualize successfully changing the one most troublesome thing. In the example of the subway, you would imagine stepping onto the train and the doors closing behind you at least 10 minutes each day and intermittently through the day. Continue for 30 days. To make this process complete, practice completing the action in real life at least two times. While doing so, recall your visualization, reminding yourself that you can do it. As you continue to practice, it becomes a habit, and you find you no longer need to remind yourself that you can do it.

This technique can also be helpful in situations such as…

- Petting a dog.
- Confidently shaking hands with an interviewer.
- Initiating a conversation with someone who intimidates you.

Visualization is a powerful tool to help change your perspective. Like automatic thoughts, you can analyze your images and change them to adopt a healthier outlook. It is often used in the treatment of anxiety disorders to help reduce symptoms and cope better with the situation. You can use imaging in combination with other CBT techniques.

# CHAPTER 7
# Relaxation Techniques and Strategies

In today's world, stress is inevitable. We spend our days rushing from one place to another. Work, family, school, and chores fill our schedules, and we barely have time to relax. This hurried and stressful lifestyle takes a physical and emotional toll. High levels of stress contribute to high blood pressure, heart disease, and digestive issues. Emotional stress shows up as irritability and anxiousness and can lead to anxiety disorders, anger problems, and depression. One part of managing stress is to learn relaxation techniques you can employ in everyday life. In this chapter, we talk about meditation and breathing techniques.

## The Importance of Breathing

We all breathe—in and out, all day, every day. Each breath we take supplies our bodies with oxygen and rids it of toxins. No matter how you breathe, you take in enough oxygen to sustain life, but often, we don't breathe properly. How you breathe affects your health, emotionally and physically. When you take in the right amount of oxygen, you give your body energy, increased focus, and feelings of relaxation and calmness. When you exhale correctly, you rid your body of harmful toxins and carbon dioxide, making room for oxygen in the blood.

Proper breathing means breathing into your chest area (allowing your ribs to get involved) and lower abdominal area (allowing your lower diaphragm to expand and contract). Both should expand when you inhale and contract on the exhale.

There are a few ways people breathe incorrectly:

*Reverse breathers* breathe into their chest on the inhale and pull their abdominal area inward and upward. Both should move together for proper breathing.

*Collapsed breathers* breathe into their lower abdominal area only and hold their chest area stationary, preventing their ribs from expanding and contracting, which can promote feelings of depression.

*Shallow breathers* breathe mostly into their chest region and hold their lower abdominal area stationary, which can cause feelings of light-headedness and anxiousness.

Many shallow breathers pull their abdomens in when breathing, forcing their shoulders upward. It makes them feel as if they are using their bellies to breathe, even though they are not. Your shoulders do not move when breathing correctly.

You can do a quick exercise to see how you breathe. Lie down with your right hand on your chest and your left hand on your abdomen. Take a few breaths, paying attention to the movement of your hands. If your right-hand moves more, you are taking shallow breathes and breathing with only the top part of your lungs. If your left-hand moves more, you are breathing mostly into your abdomen. Both hands should move together.

During periods of relaxation or sleep, you breathe slower and use more of your lungs. But during times of stress, your breathing changes, and you take more frequent shallower breaths. Quick, shallow breathing is part of the fight-or-flight response and along with an increase in adrenalin, provides a quick burst of energy to deal with an impending threat.

When facing a threat, we activate the fight-or-flight response. Our senses go on high alert to face or run from the danger. Once it passes, our bodies return to normal. That works fine when facing physical hazards, such as when our ancestors faced an animal attack or when we face a mugging. But, most of today's stresses are different; they are not a sudden attack and then a retreat. Worrying about financial problems, relationships, jobs, and security can keep you in a constant state of fight or flight. Your body stays on high alert, and your breathing continues to come in short, sharp breaths.

Proper breathing is an essential part of treatment for anxiety disorders. It also helps when managing everyday stress, chronic pain, insomnia, anger, depression, and other physical and emotional problems. The relaxation techniques in this chapter—meditation and progressive relaxation—require proper breathing to be effective.

# Your Turn: Breathing Techniques

Proper breathing takes practice. If you have been breathing improperly for years, you have conditioned your body to breathe that way; but you can retrain your body to breathe correctly. Try using one of the following exercises daily for 5 to 10 minutes. As you continue to practice, correct breathing becomes automatic.

## Feel the Difference

Lie down on the floor, with your spine straight. Place one hand on your chest and one on your abdomen. Breathe in, filling your chest, and then stop. Hold for a few seconds and then breathe out. Breathe in again, filling your belly with air. Hold for a few seconds and then release the air. Feel the difference between the two types of breathing. Understanding and feeling the difference helps you learn how to control your breathing.

## Breathe Deeply

Lie down on the floor with your knees bent, your feet slightly apart. (You can also do this sitting upright in a chair. Sit on the edge of the chair, make sure not to lean back, and keep both feet flat on the floor.) Straighten your spine. Place your right hand on your chest and your left hand on your abdomen. Inhale deeply through your nose, bringing the air into your belly. (Your left hand should rise, and your right hand should move only slightly.) Exhale through your mouth. Try to slow your breath, so you are breathing 6 to 8 times per minute. Count 4 seconds on the inhale, pause gently, and then count 4 seconds on the exhale. Pause gently before the next breath starts. Continue for 5 to 10 minutes.

## Develop Your Breathing Muscles

This exercise requires a small sandbag or 5-pound bag of rice.

Lie down on the floor with your knees bent and your feet slightly apart (about the width of your hips) and your spine straight. Place the bag of rice or the sandbag across your lower abdominal area. Relax and breathe naturally. After a few breaths, you should notice the weight of the rice causes your abdominal area to work harder during the inhale and to relax a little more on the exhale. Slow your breathing as it becomes deeper. Count 4 seconds on the inhale, pause, count 4 seconds on the exhale, pause, and then let the next deep breath begin. In this exercise, you can breathe through either your nose or your mouth, whichever feels comfortable.

## Balloon Breathing

You can do this exercise lying down or sitting upright on the edge of a chair and your feet flat on the floor. Place your right hand on your abdomen and left hand on your chest. Start by breathing slowly into your lower abdominal area and then gently inhale into your chest area (count 5 seconds). When your entire torso fills up with air like a balloon, gently hold the breath for a count of 2 to 3 seconds. When ready to exhale, purse your lips together slightly, and let the air slowly out, watching your chest and belly deflate. After fully exhaling, gently hold the abdominal area inward, count for 2 to 3 seconds and then repeat. Let the next breath begin naturally and continue this cycle. Count five-seconds for the inhale, 2 to 3 seconds to pause, 5 seconds for the exhale, and hold for 2 to 3 seconds. Repeat for 5 to 10 minutes.

## Sighing

Sighing and yawning are your body's way of getting more oxygen. You can use sighing to increase your oxygen intake and help you relax. You can do this exercise standing or sitting. Straighten your spine. Breathe in and then sigh, letting the air rush out of your lungs. Repeat several times, feeling your body relax a little more each time.

# Meditation

Meditation increases awareness and clears your mind. It's been around for a long time; the first documented reference to it goes back to India between 5000 and 3500 BCE.

Traditionally, meditation is a spiritual tool. Today, we use it to relieve stress, depression, and pain. People from all walks of life meditate daily to clear their thoughts, calm their minds, and better control their reactions to their current situation.

## What Is Meditation?

Meditation clears your mind from the barrage of constant thoughts. When meditating, you focus your thoughts on a single object (such as your breath, a photo, or an object) or a mantra (a specific word or phrase). Whenever a thought enters your mind, you bring your focus back to your object or mantra, stopping distractions from cluttering your mind. When you meditate, you are alert, yet your mind is calm.

A mantra is a sound, word, or phrase used to create a mental vibration. Mantras can have specific meanings; for example, the mantra *So Hum* means "I am." Some people repeat the sound *om* as their mantra. If you prefer using a mantra, you can choose one with a special meaning to you, use a sound, or find one from ancient meditations.

Many people find meditation difficult in the beginning. They find it hard to push aside conscious thoughts and remain quiet and still. As you practice, it becomes easier. You might even find yourself meditating for brief periods throughout the day. Some people worry that when they meditate, they lose control and fight the feeling of letting go. However, meditation is safe, and you remain aware of your surroundings.

## Why Meditate?

For centuries, monks and high priests touted the benefits of meditation, claiming it improves health, well-being, and satisfaction with life. According to recent scientific research, they could be right. Studies have shown that meditation might reduce the risk of high blood pressure, heart attack, and stroke, as well as help control chronic pain.

In addition to improving physical health, meditation has a positive effect on your emotional well-being. It lowers stress and improves symptoms of depression and anxiety. One study showed that meditating immediately before a stressful event helped participants cope better during the event. For those without specific health issues, meditation still improves empathy, compassion, and satisfaction with life.

While meditation can provide many physical and emotional benefits, it isn't right for everyone. One study found some participants reported hallucinations, panic, and a loss of motivation. Before beginning a meditation regimen, talk with your doctor. If you experience adverse effects, stop and speak with a therapist or professional who specializes in meditation.

# Your Turn: Simple Meditation

There are many different meditation techniques. The following exercise focuses on concentration. In Chapter 8, we'll go into detail on mindfulness meditation.

Before meditating, take a few minutes to stretch to help loosen your muscles and tendons, so you can sit or lie down comfortably.

*Step 1:* Find a comfortable place for your meditation. Look for somewhere peaceful and free of distractions. Turn off your phone and close your door to avoid any interruptions. While it is possible to lie down and meditate, there is a chance you could fall asleep; therefore, it is better to sit up straight in a comfortable chair or with your legs crossed on the floor while maintaining a straight back. If this is uncomfortable, try kneeling on a pillow placed on the floor.

*Step 2:* Close your eyes. Take a few moments to breathe normally, in through your nose and out through your mouth. You can take a few deep breaths to help relax if you want.

*Step 3:* Focus on your breathing. Feel your chest move up and down with each breath. Notice how your breath feels coming in and going out. Imagine yourself breathing in the goodness around you and breathing out negative thoughts.

*Step 4:* Continue to focus on your breathing. If another thought pops in your mind, simply refocus your thoughts to your breath. In the beginning, you might notice thoughts continuously popping into your head. As you practice meditation, this usually happens less often. Some people find it helpful to say "one" on the inhale, and "two" on the exhale, as it gives them a place to focus their minds. If you prefer, use a mantra, repeating it continuously.

*Step 5:* As you continue breathing, notice the stillness of your mind and relax. Continue to bring yourself back to your breathing or your mantra any time thoughts intrude.

Start with 10 to 15 minutes of meditation per day. Work your way up to about 30 minutes. If it is simpler, do two sessions of 15 minutes each. Or take time at noon to calm your mind and prepare for the rest of the day.

If you have a hard time staying focused on your breathing, consider using an app that walks you through a meditation session. When you are first starting, listening to a soothing voice that reminds you to pay attention to your breathing is sometimes helpful.

## Your Turn: Kirtan Kriya Meditation

This meditation exercise uses a simple mantra—SA TA NA MA—and stimulates your meridian points. It is an active meditation and can help those who have a hard time meditating due to distractions or an inability to relax the mind.

Meridian points are energy points in the body used in acupuncture and acupressure treatments. The belief is that stimulating these energy points improves blood circulation and stimulates nerve endings.

Research indicates this type of meditation improves memory function by increasing blood flow to vital brain structures.

*Step 1:* Sit in a chair with your feet on the floor, resisting the urge to lean back. If you prefer, you can sit on the floor cross-legged so that your ankles are touching the opposite knee. Keep your spine straight.

*Step 2:* Touch your thumb to your index finger, middle finger, ring finger, and pinky finger in sequence. As you touch each finger, vocalize one sound of the mantra (SA TA NA MA). Keep a slow, steady, and rhythmic pace.

*Step 3:* Repeat out loud for 2 minutes, repeat in a whisper for 2 minutes, and remain silent for 4 minutes. Then resume a whisper for 2 more minutes, and finally, repeat out loud for the final 2 minutes. The total time is 12 minutes.

If you have a hard time doing this on your own, there are apps for both Android and Apple to guide you through the sequence.

## Relaxing Your Muscles

Progressive muscle relaxation is a technique that involves tensing muscle groups and then relaxing them to create awareness of tension and relaxation. The term *progressive* fits because it moves through all major muscle groups, relaxing them one at a time. In the end, your entire body should feel relaxed. When your body is relaxed, your mind has calmness and clarity. Some people find it helpful to do this exercise before meditating or breathing exercises.

Many people don't even realize their muscles are tense. Progressive muscle relaxation teaches you what your muscles feel like when they are tense and when they are relaxed. Once you feel the difference, you can take a few minutes, no matter where you are, to tense and relax specific muscles to aid in reducing tension.

# Your Turn: Progressive Muscle Relaxation

Some people might find it helpful to record the instructions for this exercise and then follow along the recording. There are also apps available to lead you through progressive muscle relaxation.

Before starting, find a comfortable position. Sitting or lying down works for this exercise. Make sure you are wearing loose, comfortable clothing. Close your eyes and take a few minutes to breathe normally—in through your nose and out your mouth.

*Forehead:* Raise your eyebrows as high as possible to tighten the muscles in your forehead. Hold for 10 seconds, and then relax, feeling the release of tension.

Breathe in and out, in and out.

*Eyes:* Close your eyes tightly, holding your eyelids shut as tight as you can. Hold for 10 seconds. Release and feel your muscles loosen.

Breathe in and out, in and out.

*Mouth:* Smile as wide as you can. Tighten the muscles in your mouth and your cheeks. Hold for 10 seconds. Release, feeling your face relax and soften.

Breathe in and out, in and out.

*Head and neck:* Pull your head back as far as you can. If you are sitting, move your head as if you are looking at the ceiling. Hold for 10 seconds. Then release, feeling the muscles in your neck relax.

Let your head and neck sink back into your pillow or the back of the chair. Feel all the stress in your face and head melt away.

Breathe in and out, in and out.

*Fists:* Clench your fists, hold for 10 seconds, and release.

Breathe in and out, in and out.

*Upper Arms:* Tighten your biceps, hold for 10 seconds, and then let your muscles go limp.

Breathe in and out, in and out.

*Shoulders:* Tighten your shoulders, bringing your shoulders back as if your shoulder blades could touch. Hold for 10 seconds and release, feeling the tension in your back and shoulders dissipate.

Breathe in and out, in and out.

*Abdomen:* Tighten the muscles in your belly, sucking in air as you do. Hold for 10 seconds and release.

Allow your upper body to sink into the chair or bed, feeling the limpness in your muscles.

Breathe in and out, in and out.

*Buttocks:* Tighten your buttock muscles; hold for 10 seconds and release.

Breathe in and out, in and out.

*Thighs:* Tighten the muscles in your legs; hold for 10 seconds and release.

Breathe in and out, in and out.

*Calves:* Pull your feet toward you, feeling the muscles in your calves tighten. Hold for 10 seconds and release.

Breathe in and out, in and out.

*Toes:* Curl your toes under; hold for 10 seconds and release.

Let your legs sink into your mattress or chair. Feel how relaxed your muscles are.

Breathe in and out, in and out.

As with meditation, this exercise takes practice. The first few times you complete the activity, you might not notice much difference. Be patient and continue to practice progressive muscle relaxation every day. As you practice, it becomes easier to control your muscles.

# Other Ways to Relax

With all your responsibilities, it might be challenging to find time for hobbies, socializing, and exercise, especially if you feel overwhelmed. However, not giving yourself time to unwind can be harmful to your health. As much as possible, allow yourself time to relax and take pleasure in life. When it seems there isn't enough time, remind yourself it is essential for your physical and emotional well-being.

## Hobbies

A hobby can be anything. The Oxford Dictionary defines it as "an activity done regularly in one's leisure time for pleasure." The key here is to do it regularly. Hobbies are great for relaxation and lowering stress, but only if you make time for them. No matter what you like to do—fishing, dancing, reading, biking, canoeing, gardening, or painting, schedule 1 hour a week to participate in activities you enjoy.

If you've been neglecting a hobby that you enjoy, reintroduce it into your life. You might tell yourself you will get back to your pastime when your children are grown, when your job is less demanding, or when you have more time. Life might never slow down, so it's crucial to find time now.

# Your Turn: Create a Wish List

*The form accompanying this exercise is in Appendix C.*

Write down activities you enjoy that help you relax. Think back over the past and include hobbies or activities you once enjoyed, even if you haven't participated for a long time. Include things you want to learn. You created a hobby bucket list.

Put a star next to one or two activities high on your list of "wants." Be creative in scheduling time each day or week to submerge yourself in your hobbies. The trick is finding a way to build activities you enjoy into your schedule. Consider these strategies:

- Wake up a half-hour earlier than usual and give yourself quiet time to pursue an interest.
- Trade evenings with your partner. One evening a week, you oversee the household and kids; the other is your partner's turn. Use your one night a week to pursue activities you enjoy.
- If possible, take advantage of flex time at work. Add a half-hour to your day two days a week, and then leave an hour early one day to focus on you.
- Use your lunch hour one day a week to do something you enjoy.

Think about what prevented you from doing the activities on your wish list and create a response plan. Pay attention to what gets in the way of achieving your goals and develop a plan of action to combat excuses and reasons.

Hobbies are fun and enjoyable but should not overtake your life; work toward a balance. Everyone's lifestyle and responsibilities are different—what works for one person could be too little or too much time for another. Find the amount of time each day or week that works for you and make it a priority.

## Social Activities

Getting together with friends and family to enjoy their company is essential. Research shows people with strong social connections are better able to manage stress, are healthier, and live longer than those who lead solitary lives.

As teens and young adults, social activities are a big part of our lives. But as we get older, work and family become more demanding. As years pass, your partner and your children might become your sole social outlet. However, having a social network is essential to well-being. Friends fill in the gaps and give you someone to talk to, to share stories with, and to ask for (and give) help.

If you are having a hard time finding friends outside of your family and coworkers, consider the following ideas.

**Look for adult classes in your area.** Use the wish list you created in the last exercise to search for interesting courses, a great way to meet people with similar interests.

**Sign up for classes at an alternative gym.** Traditional gyms don't provide much opportunity for socializing. However, there are alternative exercise options that allow you to be with people who like the same thing as you, such as yoga classes, rock climbing, or pole dancing.

**Join a group.** Websites such as Facebook and Meetup have groups for just about any interest. Local businesses are also an excellent resource; for example, specialty stores such as yarn shops, home-brewing supply stores, and bookstores often host monthly get-togethers.

**Use social media sites.** Websites such as Instagram give you the opportunity to meet people with similar interests. Following local Instagram pages can lead to in-person and virtual events.

**Look for community events.** Another way to meet people is to attend local events such as races, fundraisers, and festivals. Some are family affairs that welcome children and pets, which makes them a great way to meet other parents with children about the same age. You can also volunteer and meet people behind the scenes.

**Visit a place of worship.** Many churches, temples, mosques, and synagogues offer an array of groups, workshops, and events in addition to weekly services.

**Volunteer.** Seek out organizations in your area based on your interests and passions. Check with the local hospital, senior center, or parks department. Volunteer to spend time with the animals at a local pet shelter. If you want to take small steps, start by volunteering to help at a one-time event and work your way up to volunteering weekly.

## Physical Activity and Exercise Programs

We know exercise is good for our physical health. It improves how the body functions, decreases anxiety and depression, and improves sleep, concentration, and cognitive function. Between the ages of 19 and 64, you should get at least 150 minutes of exercise per week.

# Your Turn: Activity Journal

*The form accompanying this exercise is in Appendix C.*

How often do you do physical activities? Not just traditional exercise or going to the gym, but how often do you do actions that get your body moving? Exercise doesn't necessarily mean going to "work out" on the treadmill or weight machines. You might exercise more often than you think you do.

Create an activity journal by keeping track of your activity on a computer, paper, a fitness bracelet, or by using an activity tracking app. Record times for any activity you did that day. Maybe you walked in the mall for an hour, did some gardening, took the steps instead of the elevator, took your kids swimming, or played golf. Keeping track of these types of activities might motivate you to do more. At the end of the week, review your accomplishments and set goals for the following week. The purpose of this activity is not to become physically fit but to increase movement.

## Create a Fitness Program

The first step to creating a fitness program is deciding when you are going to exercise. It's easy to say, "I'll walk 3 miles each day," but that also makes it easy to not to have time one day and not have time again the next day until you stop completely. Instead, commit and set aside a specific time each day, even if you start with 10 minutes a day.

Research on patients who underwent hip surgery showed those who made a specific action plan were significantly more likely to exercise and recovered more quickly than those who said they would walk 20 minutes a day. For example, "I will meet my partner at the bus stop after work and walk home together."

Structure your exercise time. You might go to the gym and do a specific set of exercises, join a weekly class, or commit to a routine or workout video at home. Using the right structured program for your needs and your level helps you stick to the plan.

You also need to set goals. Setting goals gives you a purpose for exercising. Are you trying to lose weight? Be more physically fit? Increase your energy? You need to know what to look for to see progress. Setting specific goals not only gives you something to work toward, but it gives you a way to know when you get there. Create a physical goal, such as walking for 20 minutes daily.

Set a specific action plan, such as, "I will walk home from the train station every day" or "I will spend the second half of my lunch hour walking around the building." Then create an outcome goal. What is one measurable thing? Track and record your progress daily or weekly. If you find it challenging to set goals, review Chapter 5. An example of an action plan is:

## Specific Action Plan

| Date | Action Goal | Action Plan | Outcome Goal |
| --- | --- | --- | --- |
| 9/19 | Walk 20 min. | Walk from train | Weight = 154 lbs |
| 9/26 | Walk 30 min. | Walk to and from the train | Weight = 152 lbs |

Relaxation strategies are a great way to lower stress and improve physical health. Learning to breathe correctly is vital; strive for deep breathing, using your chest and abdomen. Meditation and progressive muscle relaxation both require correct breathing. Other relaxation strategies, such as exercise, hobbies, and social activities, are essential for you to maintain a sense of well-being.

# CHAPTER 8
# Mindfulness

When you practice mindfulness, you live in the moment; it helps you look at your thought process—not to change it, but to observe without judgment. While different from many of the traditional CBT techniques, it still plays an integral part in understanding and changing behaviors. In this chapter, you learn what mindfulness is and how to incorporate it into daily life.

## What Is Mindfulness?

According to the Oxford Dictionary, mindfulness is "a mental state achieved by focusing one's awareness on the present moment, while calmly acknowledging and accepting one's feelings, thoughts and bodily sensations." It teaches you to focus on the present and to remove yourself from the past and future. When you practice mindfulness, you simply observe and feel without analyzing or contemplating your thoughts or the environment. It is accepting what is happening right now, without thinking about whether it is right or wrong or looking for solutions. Mindfulness is a way of being rather than doing.

Your brain's autopilot tends to default to doing mode. You assess for discrepancies between what is happening and what you think should happen (or should have happened). Your brain's autopilot is sometimes harmful, especially if you are prone to worrying and depression, because it often leads to rumination. Mindfulness exercises enhance your brain's ability to utilize and benefit from the being mode of the mind.

Rumination is the mental act of reviewing and analyzing thoughts and situations repeatedly, including why you feel the way you do. When ruminating, you attempt to answer the self-imposed question, "Why?" For example, suppose you were in a car accident. You might relive the minutes leading up to the accident to see if you could have done something to avoid it (even if the accident is deemed to not be your fault). You relive those moments repeatedly, sometimes for days or weeks. The problem with rumination is it frequently brings up similar memories to validate your thoughts. In the car accident example, you might decide you were distracted, which contributed to the accident. Your mind automatically remembers other times you were distracted, reinforcing your idea that you are at fault. Ruminations tend to be negative; if you are fearful of having another car accident, you recall the collision and any near misses you had. You ignore the thousands of times you drove without an accident. Mindfulness prevents rumination by bringing you back to the present moment.

## Your Turn: Mindfulness Breathing

Many people begin practicing mindfulness by focusing on their breathing, such as using traditional meditation practices. Unlike them, you can be mindful while engaging with the world. The purpose of the exercise is to train your mind to focus on one element of your present experience.

Find a comfortable, quiet area and sit upright. You can keep your eyes open or closed, whichever you find more relaxing.

Listen to the sound of your breath without changing your breathing. How does it sound on the inhale and the exhale? Do you make a sound during the moments in between your inhale and exhale? Notice how it feels when air enters your nose, notice how it feels as you fill your chest and abdomen with air, and notice the sensations as you exhale. Pay attention to each breath, from the moment you start to inhale until the moment the air leaves your body.

Continue for 10 minutes. Each time you notice your thoughts wandering, take notice, and bring your attention back to your breathing. Don't judge yourself for letting your attention wander, and don't analyze the feeling. Simply notice that you had a thought and return to paying attention to your breathing.

Practice this exercise once a day for a week. As you do, you should notice your thoughts wandering less often and your attention on your breath with greater ease.

## A Thought Is Just a Thought

You can more easily move on to other thoughts when you observe and accept a negative thought or emotion without reacting to it. In other words, you allow a negative impression to exist without fixating on it or giving it any weight. Your attitude becomes "It is just a thought," and you know not all thoughts are reliable or permanent. Once you accept the "just a thought" perspective, the idea no longer has any hold on you.

Imagine you are waiting for a call from a potential client. You think, "He is not going to call; I lost the sale." Your mind has a few choices. You can ruminate on the idea, remembering every sale you lost, or you can accept that it is just a thought and that thinking something doesn't make it true. Instead of ruminating on the idea or testing its validity, you let it go. You move on, focusing on the work you are doing right now.

## The Role of Mindfulness in CBT

Many of the techniques and strategies used in CBT work to change your thoughts and behaviors; mindfulness, although frequently used in CBT, works differently. It's not about challenging ideas; instead, it's about accepting that a thought exists without needing further attention. In mindfulness, you use thought distancing—you don't try to change, analyze, prove, disprove, or interact with it. You simply accept you had it. The more you learn to distance, the more you let things go. You don't spend unnecessary time analyzing information that doesn't matter. Distancing helps you gain control of your thoughts. By allowing yourself to see thoughts and feelings without judgment and analysis, you reduce the tendency to relapse into ruminations.

Mindfulness gives you space to pause and prioritize the issues you want to address. In the example of waiting for a call, if you didn't practice mindfulness, you could have invested unnecessary energy into a fleeting thought.

Unproductive thought processes frequently follow one of two paths. One is to feed into it, creating an entire narrative to back up your negative thought. In the previous example, suppose you focused on, "He is not going to call; I lost the sale." You continue chaining negative thoughts until you have worked yourself into a frenzy. The second path is to attempt to avoid negative thinking—pushing it from your mind. You tell yourself that you don't want to have that thought, which rarely works. Mindfulness provides a third option. It allows you to see and accept the negative thinking and then move on because "it's just a thought." Think of it as watching television. You are engrossed in a show, and when a commercial airs, you tune it out. You know it is there, but it is "just a commercial." When the show returns, you are once again engrossed and no longer think about the commercial.

## Controlling Urges

In the beginning, you might notice it is tough to see a thought, feeling, or urge without responding to it. Practicing mindfulness helps you accept challenging emotions and impulses without acting every time. For example, suppose you want to lose weight. While in a restaurant, you order a salad. Then, the dessert tray goes by. You have a strong urge to order chocolate cake for dessert. You can give in and get a piece, or you can accept the feeling without giving in to it. An urge is nothing more than a thought with a request for action. You can acknowledge and then dismiss it as you do with other thoughts. You can resist acting on it. When you first start practicing mindfulness, you might become frustrated because you can't stop unwanted thoughts or distractions. Be persistent and keep trying. As with anything, mindfulness takes commitment and practice. The longer you work at it, the easier it becomes, and the more you realize the benefits.

## Your Turn: The Raisin Experience

This exercise is an excellent way to practice mindfulness. You focus on the raisin and the experience of eating the raisin to develop your ability to be mindful.

Place a raisin in your hand. Look at it. Examine how it feels in your hand. Notice the smell, texture, and color of the raisin. Lay the raisin on your tongue. Close your eyes. Notice again how the raisin feels. Notice how it tastes as it lies on your tongue. Notice your urge to eat the raisin. Just notice them. Don't give in to the desire to eat the raisin. Just notice how it feels. Then, after one minute, start to chew the raisin. Notice every sensation as you chew. Don't swallow. Notice the urge without giving in. After one minute, swallow the raisin. Notice any bodily changes as you consume the raisin, including the changes in facial, hand, and body muscles. Notice the differences in muscle tension in your face and throat after you swallow the raisin. Notice any thoughts and sensations after swallowing the raisin.

Your goal is to become wholly immersed in the experience of eating a raisin.

## Being Present in the Moment

Today is the only important day; this moment is a single critical moment. You have heard this before. Even so, you probably spend most of your time thinking about what happened yesterday and worrying about what might happen tomorrow. Though you are living this moment, you are not present in it—unless you focus on it.

You might wonder how it is possible, or even helpful, to live only in this moment. After all, you have goals and dreams for your future. If you live in this moment, how can you take the steps needed to reach your goals? How can you plan? The confusion is in understanding what mindfulness is and what it isn't. When you are mindful, you are conscious of your thoughts—the thoughts you have at this moment. But they can be thoughts about the future. Mindfulness is focused thinking, not daydreaming; you can be mindful about the past or the future.

When planning, ask yourself:

> What do I want to happen?
>
> What steps do I need to get there?

When thinking about the past, ask yourself:

> What can I learn from this experience to help me grow?

Mindfulness is about your thoughts in the present moment, but those thoughts don't need to be about the present moment. The exercises in this chapter introduce the concept of mindfulness and teach you how to focus your thoughts. Once you can do that, you can use mindfulness in any aspect of your life.

Practicing mindfulness helps you incorporate it into different parts of your life, including times when you face challenging or uncomfortable situations. There are times in your life when you anticipate feeling uncomfortable. Be mindful of yourself and what is happening around you. Ask "What do I want, and how do I get there?" to help you distance yourself and cope more easily.

Suppose you are afraid of flying and are about to board an airplane. Instead of worrying about all the possible disasters and thinking that you can't handle being on a plane (daydreaming), try focusing on your body's sensations. Notice each thought that passes through your mind (mindfulness). Identify thoughts about uncertainty and those about your discomfort. Remind yourself that "These are just thoughts. Thinking them does not make them true." You should begin to feel grounded and more in control of your emotions and better equipped to manage the situation.

A quick exercise for refocusing unwanted thoughts is to stop and notice your surroundings. What do you see? What do you smell? Use all five senses to take in your surroundings. Notice how your clothes feel. What do you hear? Notice if you are hot, cold, or comfortable. Note if you are relaxed or tense. What are your points of tension? Take some deep breaths and feel the tension leaving every time you exhale. Pay attention to what is happening at this very moment, which should help you to feel calmer and in a better position to look at your situation objectively.

## Tips for Living in the Present Moment

*Spend 10 minutes a day practicing mindfulness.* Pick a necessary task that you do mindlessly, such as brushing your teeth or washing dishes. In each of these experiences, pay attention to all five senses. Notice any thoughts and emotions. Just notice without reacting. The more you practice, the more you will find yourself stopping throughout the day to appreciate the moment.

*Don't rush.* When you hurry through a task, you are probably more focused on what comes next than the moment at hand. Use slow, deliberate movements. As you put more focus on each task, you find they are more satisfying.

*Reduce activities that don't promote mindfulness.* Turn off the television, shut off your phone. Eliminate whatever distracts you from paying attention to the moment. If you find yourself reacting negatively to the people around you and what they are doing, focus on accepting them for how they choose to behave. Instead of judging their actions as "wrong," just notice your thoughts and body sensations.

*Take the time to be present in conversations.* Listen to what the other person is saying and respond thoughtfully. Don't rush to express your own opinions.

## Watch Your Thoughts Sail By

To help you see thoughts without judging them, think of them as sailboats. Instead of trying to fix them, just notice them sailing by. When sitting by the sea, it is pleasurable to watch boats sail across the water. When you have an unfocused or negative thought, imagine placing it on the sailboat and watching as it navigates out of sight. Remember, thoughts are not good or bad; they simply are. You can recognize that you feel sad, frustrated, or angry, but know the feeling will pass and that it is temporary. As you practice watching your thoughts sail by, think, "I am angry, but this is a passing thought, and I will get through it."

## Your Turn: Observing Thoughts

Sit back in a comfortable chair, with your back upright. Spend a few minutes focused on your breathing; pay attention to how your breath feels as it enters your body, fills your abdomen, and then leaves your body. Don't change your breathing; just notice it. Then turn your attention to your thoughts, recognizing they are simply thoughts. Place them on the boat and let them go. Do not make any judgments; just notice them.

Use this technique daily to help gather information about what is on your mind and gain a sense of your autopilot mode. You are practicing "being" rather than "doing," which helps build mental flexibility, allowing you to direct your attention as needed. The point of this exercise is to let your thoughts happen and to better understand your unconscious mind.

## Accepting Upsetting Thoughts and Moods

**When feeling sad, upset, or angry, you might try to analyze your thoughts by asking yourself:**

- Why do I feel this way?
- What did I do to cause this feeling?
- Did I act differently than I usually do?
- What other times have I felt this way?

You probably ask these questions to feel better, but analyzing your thoughts often leads to ruminating—remembering past times you were sad and angry or blaming yourself or others. As you delve into answers about your mood, you frequently feel worse.

Instead of "solving" your mood, try accepting it, and all it encompasses, including physical sensations. For example, when you are anxious, you might have a racing heart, shortness of breath, an upset stomach, or you might be trembling. When noticing your thought, stop to pay attention to your body's reaction and any sensations you feel. Pay attention to changes in your body and your thoughts as the emotion flows through you. Your feelings can ebb and flow. For example, you might feel sad for a little while; then, as your thoughts change, the sadness might disappear only to return later.

Try to describe the facts of what you're feeling.

- My stomach feels like it is in knots.
- I have a headache.
- I feel sad.
- I am having a hard time breathing.

Writing down thoughts and accompanying sensations in a factual way helps you create distance. You are separating emotions and facts; you acknowledge thoughts are part of the process rather than the process itself.

In the beginning, you might use mindfulness mostly when having negative thoughts and experiences. But mindfulness can be used in every aspect of your life. For example, you can use it to focus on gratefulness.

# Incorporating Mindfulness in Everyday Life

Mindfulness practice sessions give you an overall sense of well-being, and it is essential to incorporate them into daily life. But don't leave mindfulness in your chair. There are plenty of opportunities throughout your day to be mindful.

*While brushing your teeth.* Pay attention to the taste of your toothpaste in your mouth and how it smells. Notice how the toothbrush feels going across your teeth; be mindful of each tooth. Notice the sound of the toothbrush as you brush your teeth. Pay attention to how your arms move. Ignore the urge to look in the mirror, check your hair, or multitask while getting ready for work. Pay attention to only the task of brushing your teeth.

*Waiting in line.* In our hectic lives, there are usually times throughout the day when you wait in line—waiting for lunch, buying groceries, sitting in traffic, or being on hold. You see this as wasted time and frustrating; you want to get done and get back to your routine. Waiting for something stops you from doing other things. Instead of becoming impatient, take the time to breathe deeply. Pay attention to where in your body you feel tense. Instead of focusing on frustration, use this time as an opportunity to be quiet and still for a few moments.

*Eating.* Enjoy the entire process of eating. Notice how the food looks on your plate and the different colors and textures. Pay attention to the smell of the food. Savor each bite, noticing the texture, temperature, and taste. Notice how the silverware feels in your hand. Pay attention to those around you, and focus on what they are saying.

*Taking a shower.* Pay attention to how the water feels on your body and how the soap or shower gel smells and feels. Feel the temperature of the water. Listen to how it sounds as it hits your body and the walls of the shower. Notice the feel of the shower floor on your feet.

No matter how hectic your day is, you can find time to be mindful. Stop several times during the day to pause for a few minutes, take several deep breaths, and be in the present moment. Write down five things you notice at this moment, one for each of the senses. A 5 minute mindfulness break can leave you feeling refreshed and connected to your environment.

# Your Turn: Diary of Mindfulness Exercises

The exercises introduced in this chapter are excellent ways to start practicing mindfulness every day. Before you know it, it becomes a habit.

Keep a journal of your mindfulness exercises. Record the following for each one you do:

- Date.
- Mindfulness activity.
- Location.
- On a scale of 1 to 10, how easy it was for you to be mindful?
- Were you were distracted?
- One word to describe what you observed during your mindfulness activity.
- One word to describe how you felt when done.

During times of stress, you might find it harder to be mindful. Instead of judging yourself as a failure or retreating to bad habits, accept this as a part of stress. You'll find it becomes more comfortable with time.

Mindfulness is focusing on the present moment and acknowledging your thoughts without judgment. Doing so helps you separate facts from emotion and allows you to view a situation more objectively. The practice of mindfulness reduces symptoms of anxiety and depression by focusing on the here and now, rather than worrying about the past or the future. When you are mindful, you accept that thoughts come and go, and something isn't true just because you think it. An easy way to practice mindfulness is to stop and pay attention to what you are experiencing by focusing on your five senses.

# CHAPTER 9
# Your Inner Narration

Your inner voice talks to you every day. It tells you what you do right and what you do wrong. Even when you don't like what it says, it is impossible to turn off. In this chapter, we discuss how to change the words and tone of your inner voice, recognize and respond to internal criticisms, and replace those criticisms with more positive perspectives.

## Self-Talk

As you go through your day, your thoughts continually churn in your head. Your inner voice narrates everything that happens, guiding you and your decisions. Sometimes, it is positive: "I am getting a raise;" sometimes, it is neutral: "I need to call my client to reschedule the missed meeting;" sometimes, it is negative: "This meeting is not going well."

Generally, there are three ways you internally narrate what is happening around you:

*Situational:* You describe a situation, including your expectations, assumptions, and opinions.

*Others:* You create opinions and judgments based on what you expect from others.

*Me:* You make judgments and assumptions about yourself based on your core beliefs.

Typically, you believe everything your inner voice tells you. Most of the time, you don't bother to double check or fact-check the information. You approach situations based on whether your inner voice is positive, negative, or neutral.

*Negative:* When your inner voice is negative, you approach the world in a closed-off, impatient, or cynical way. Your self-talk might center around sentiments like, "I am going to fail," "People are selfish," or "The world is a bad place." When you assume the worst in yourself and others, it is hard to find solutions to problems. You are frequently angry or irritable.

*Positive:* When you have optimistic self-talk, you approach the world with the belief that "I can handle this," "Someone will help me," or "There is a solution to this problem." You believe the glass is half full," and you are usually optimistic.

*Neutral:* When your inner voice is mostly neutral, you approach situations with a matter-of-fact attitude. You see occurrences as neither positive or negative; you might think, "I have a busy day," but you don't attach an opinion or perspective to your statement. You are usually open to whatever comes along.

Inner talk is frequently in the form of short sentences or phrases rather than full sentences, such as "Great," "Now what?" or "Oh, no." When you have positive or neutral self-talk, you are more likely to approach life with curiosity, openness, and tolerance.

Most of the time, you don't notice these thoughts; they automatically happen as you do your job, take care of your children, relate to your spouse, run errands, and so on. You might think about the "big picture," but you don't necessarily pay attention to how you narrate the small moments of your day. Although you might lean toward one type of narration, you probably bounce from one to the other, depending on the situation.

# Your Turn: Recording Your Inner Dialogue

*The form accompanying this exercise is in Appendix C.*

The first step to changing negative self-talk is to listen to how you narrate your life.

Over the next day or two, set the alarm to signal you every hour. When the alarm goes off, take 5 minutes to review the past hour; note what is going on around you and note your thoughts. Determine if your inner narration was positive, negative, or neutral. Try to sum up your emotion for the hour in one word.

Example:

> 9:00 A.M.—10:00 A.M.
>
> My spouse and I went grocery shopping. My spouse watched the cash register like a hawk, paying attention to every price, and stopping the cashier when he thought there was a discrepancy. This forced the cashier to stop ringing up the groceries and answer his question, even though the prices she rang up were always correct. The people in line behind us became visibly annoyed because ringing up our groceries took much longer than it should have. I was annoyed and embarrassed. I thought my spouse was overly hawkish with the grocery bill and insensitive to the people in line behind us. I acted very abruptly with my spouse.
>
> Inner narration: Negative
>
> Emotional rating: Annoyed, almost angry

If your inner narration was cynical, think about how you could change it to neutral or positive. For example, you might change your narrative to observe your spouse's behavior but without adding in your perspective or judgment.

# Types of Negative Narrations

Negative narrations usually fall into one of four categories. Read the following profiles to see which one sounds most like your inner dialogue.

## The Worrier

The theme behind your thoughts is "What if…?" This type of self-talk can lead to anxiety or depression. You might…

- Anticipate worst-case outcomes.
- Overestimate the odds that something harmful or embarrassing will happen.
- Underestimate the possibility that things will turn out okay.

As soon as you realize you are worrying about something, ask yourself five questions:

- Is this situation as bad as I imagine it to be?
- What is the worst that could happen?
- What is the best that could happen?
- What is most likely to happen?
- How important is this going to be in 5 years?

Often, taking the time to look at the situation from different perspectives calms worrying.

Your inner voice is always on guard, ready to point out anything wrong. Problematic thinking processes for the worrier include catastrophizing, overgeneralizing, and fortune-telling.

Some examples include…

- My heart is racing; it must be a heart attack.
- This is hard. I am going to fail.
- Things will never improve.

Even when things go well, you are skeptical. You don't believe it will last or don't think you deserve the good fortune.

## Self-Critique

This type of inner dialogue breeds low self-esteem. The underlying theme is, "I am not good enough." It contributes to not meeting personal goals because as soon as you make a mistake or hit a snag, you give up. You make excuses to avoid trying.

A few examples include…

- That was stupid; I can't believe I did it.
- I already cheated on my diet; I might as well eat the cake.
- I won't ever be as capable as they are.

The critic inside your head consistently judges what you do and say. You are quick to point out faults and limitations. When you narrate your world this way, you remind yourself of past failures and compare yourself to others, always coming up short. Problematic thought processes include discounting the positive, self-blaming, and overgeneralizing.

## The Victim/Blamer

This type of inner voice leads to hopelessness and helplessness. The theme is "I can't," "I will never be able to," or "It's my fault."

Some examples include…

- I'll never be able to do that. Why bother trying?".
- I am hopeless.
- This wouldn't have happened if I….

Problematic thought processes for this type of narration include blaming others and catastrophizing.

When your self-talk includes problematic thinking styles of "blame" or "should" toward others, you don't take any personal responsibility.

## The Perfectionist

You criticize your abilities and push yourself to do better. This inner voice lets you know you aren't trying hard enough or doing enough. You tell yourself, "I should have" or "I must." It comes from the part of you that wants to be the best but doesn't tolerate mistakes or failures. It convinces you that self-worth comes from external sources, not from within you.

Examples include...

- I should always be the best.
- I must always complete my goals.
- Any setback is a failure.

When the perfectionist takes over, you push yourself into high levels of stress and exhaustion. The problematic thinking patterns include "should" and "must".

## Checklist for More Positive Inner Narration

After you identify negativity in your inner narration, you can reword your thoughts. The following questions might help:

*Is my thought specific or general?*

Create statements specific to individuals or situations. For example, rather than "I don't get along with my colleagues," say, "Tom and I do not agree all the time." Be as specific as possible.

*Is my thought flexible or stable?*

Consider situations can change. Instead of "I am not good at my job," you can say, "With some additional training, I can complete this task." Focus on how situations can change and improve with time, effort, or assistance.

*Is my thought external or personal?*

Create statements that are neutral or external rather than making events and situations about you. Instead of saying, "Every other lawn on my street looks so much better than mine," say, "Lawn and garden work is not my strong suit, but I am good at...."

*Is my thought about what I can control or about what isn't working?*

Change your focus to what you can control within a situation rather than what is wrong with it. Instead of saying, "My coworkers don't want to talk to me," say, "I can start a conversation with someone."

## Your Turn: Which Category?

*The form accompanying this exercise in is Appendix C.*

Pay attention to how you talk to yourself. When you notice cynical narration, stop, and go through the following steps:

1. Place your thought into one of these categories: worrier, self-critique, victim/blamer, or perfectionist.

2. Identify the problematic thought process you used.

3. Come up with a new neutral or positive thought.

For example, suppose you got home from work late and rather than preparing dinner, you ordered a pizza. You might think, "I am so lazy."

*Category:* perfectionist, self-critique

*Problematic Thought Processes:* labeling, overgeneralization

New thought: "I work hard. Getting take-out occasionally is fine."

# Affirmations

Inner dialogue reflects beliefs, many of which you learned in childhood. Some are no longer relevant in your life. You can use affirmations to help change these to more appropriate and positive ways of looking at yourself, your life, and the world around you. Affirmations are a choice to think positive thoughts.

Change isn't always easy. Imagine you have a hard time making friends, and because of that, you only have one friend. You believe you are unlovable. You have probably carried this belief for many years. Create a positive affirmation, such as "I am a lovable person. I can make new friends" is going to be hard for you to say. At first, you don't believe it, and you might feel intense resistance. Your subconscious finds it easier and more comfortable to hold onto the old belief.

Continually repeating your affirmation and stating it aloud with conviction, slowly chips away at your resistance. The more often you say it, the more you begin to live and behave as if it is true. You are challenging negative beliefs and replacing them with a more positive inner truth. Positive affirmations reprogram your thoughts and acting on them helps you see yourself more positively. Small changes add up to significant changes.

# Combating the Idea of Lying to Yourself

Suppose you are shy. You avoid social gatherings because they make you uncomfortable, and you usually end up standing by yourself. You decide to use positive affirmations to help you feel more comfortable. First, write down your negative thoughts:

When I go to a social gathering, I feel rejected. I have a hard time talking to people and starting conversations, so I sit or stand by myself off to the side and feel like no one wants to talk to me. Because of that, I avoid social gatherings.

And write down a positive affirmation:

> I am an intelligent and thoughtful person with many experiences I can share with others. People I know enjoy my company. I can start conversations and talk to other people confidently.

As you repeat this statement every day, you have a nagging feeling you are lying to yourself. After a few days, you give up. You know you don't feel comfortable at social gatherings; you think telling yourself you do feel comfortable is not going to help, so you give up. Your subconscious rejected the affirmation.

## Making Affirmations Believable

It helps if you soften your affirmation to make it more believable. You might start with, "Meeting new people can be fun and interesting." To back this up, think about other times you have enjoyed meeting someone and found the conversation interesting. Now, you have a statement you can believe. Start with this statement every day. Because you have already thought about evidence to back it up, your subconscious should not reject it. As you repeat it each day, you might start looking forward to meeting new people and seek opportunities when you can do so.

Sometimes, it helps to listen to your arguments with yourself. If you tell yourself, "I like meeting new people," an automatic thought might pop up, reminding you that you are not interesting. You talk yourself out of believing the affirmation. When this occurs, combat your automatic negative thought with a new affirmation; in this case, it might be, "I am interesting to talk to because…."

If repeating and believing affirmations is still difficult, try adding words such as *choose* or *potential* to make them more believable. You might say, "I have the potential to be interesting," or "I choose to meet new people." These words signal a willingness to improve and change, and they give you a sense of empowerment because you know things can be different in the future.

## Seeing the Big Picture

For some people, seeing the big picture and making affirmations that reflect their final goal works. You imagine what it is you want and then change your narration to tell yourself you are already there. It is the "fake it until you make it" mindset. Your mind doesn't know the difference between reality and make-believe, so if you tell it something often enough, it accepts it as accurate. Affirmations are a way of telling yourself what you want to believe and repeating those things often.

Some people have trouble with this approach and end up feeling worse because they are making things up. They repeat the affirmation every day, but the automatic thoughts tell them, "This is a lie." If this happens, try breaking the affirmation into small pieces and work on a small change until the little changes add up to the big picture.

# Tips for Creating Affirmations

How you word your affirmations makes the difference between being helpful and causing distress. The following are tips to help create effective affirmations:

*Start your affirmation with "I am" rather than "I want."* Using the present tense increases the feeling that you already have something. (This is particularly helpful when using personal traits, such as outgoing, engaging, competent.) Using the words "I want" can leave you feeling as if you are inadequate because you don't already have the trait.

*Write affirmations in a positive tone.* Don't write what you want to avoid or what you want to eliminate. Write based on what you want to have or gain. For example, don't say, "I don't want to get distressed about finances all the time." Instead, say, "I have a comfortable life."

*Use counterstatements to create affirmations to dispute automatic thoughts.* For example, say, "I am a hard worker," if you usually tell yourself you are lazy.

*Write down your affirmations.* The act of writing them down reinforces them.

*Keep affirmations short.* Remembering one sentence is much easier than remembering a paragraph.

*Include evidence in your affirmation.* If you find your automatic thoughts outweigh your assertion, try starting with evidence; for example, say "I am friends with Chris; therefore, I can make friends."

*Make affirmations about yourself.* You can't change other people and repeating how you want others to change is not going to work. Your statements should be about ways you want to improve your life.

*Avoid ambiguous words or comparatives.* Keep affirmations specific. Don't say, "I am going to be a better person." Instead, say, "I am a good listener."

Changing your inner thoughts takes time. Be patient and continue repeating your affirmations.

Self-talk is your inner dialogue. You use it to narrate and interpret your experiences, and you can do so positively, negatively, or in a neutral way. Negative self-talk could manifest as worry, self-criticism, self-blame, and perfectionism. Noticing how you talk to yourself and changing the negative narration to reflect a positive, balanced perspective improves feelings of self-worth and well-being.

# CHAPTER 10
# Testing Your New Beliefs

In CBT, reality testing provides a way to test old thoughts and beliefs and reinforce new ideas. It compares how you previously thought to new beliefs so you can decide which are more helpful. The preceding chapters helped you become aware of your thoughts, analyze them, find the negative thought processes, and come up with alternative views and beliefs. In this chapter, you go one step further by creating experiments to test out new beliefs and thinking styles. In essence, you learn to test your new reality.

## Reality Testing

As you complete thought logs, you discover different ways of thinking. They might make sense, but you might not be convinced. You might need proof before accepting a new way of thinking about yourself, others, and the world. Reality testing, also called *behavioral experiments*, allows you to be interactive in the CBT process. It is a set of concrete actions that seek to prove your new way of thinking and disprove your old way of thinking.

To create a behavioral experiment, start with your ABCD log:

**A:** Describe the situation and identify a problem.

**B:** Record negative beliefs.

**C:** Record what you assume will happen.

**D:** Identify problematic thought processes (see Chapter 2). Write down ideas to challenge these views.

Now add column E (evidence testing) and create an experiment to test out your predictions and beliefs.

Write down your desired outcome. Consider other ways the situation could develop. Record how much you believe in this new outcome, using a scale of 0 to 100 percent.

Once you complete the chart, create an action plan to test your new outcome. Include specific actions to increase the chances of your desired outcome occurring. For example, suppose a friend invites you to a picnic. You are nervous because you don't know anyone besides the host. Your original thought is "I won't fit in with their friends." Your desired outcome is "to find at least one person I feel comfortable talking with, and I think there is a 60 percent chance this will happen. My specific steps are smile and say hello to at least five people, and ask questions about their interests." Go to the picnic and put your plan into action. Afterward, write down what happened and then review the information. Ask yourself…

> On a scale of 1 to 100 percent, how close did I follow the plan?
>
> On a scale of 1 to 100 percent, how close was the outcome for your new prediction?

When reviewing the results, try to look at them from a positive perspective. Pay attention to your thoughts; if you notice negative thinking patterns, come up with positive ways to look at the situation. Review the skills in Chapters 1 and 2 to help you view the results more objectively. Reality testing should reinforce new beliefs and give you a reason to continue making changes in your thinking and behavior.

The following is an example of reality testing:

**A:** You are attending a party.

**B:** You predict you won't know many people. You anticipate it will be a disaster. You think you will feel left out and that others will find you uninteresting.

**C:** You are anxious and don't want to go to the party.

**D:** I am overgeneralizing and fortune-telling about all parties and all people. After all, the person who invited me is a nice person. I do not have any information to prove the people at the party will reject me. I have been in new situations before, and they turned out okay. If I am not enjoying myself, I can leave after an hour. I do not have any evidence that I am not capable of holding a conversation with others or successfully attending a party.

**E:** I can go to the party for at least one hour and talk with at least two people. This will prove I can navigate a party successfully.

Behavior Plan/Strategy:

- Bring a bottle of wine and thank my host for inviting me.
- Make small talk with a few guests.

- Smile and say hello to everyone.
- Ask other guests questions, such as "Where do you work?" and "What do you like to do on the weekends?"

Once you create a plan, do your best to follow through. Then review and rate the results. For example:

I would give an overall outcome rating of 80 percent because I enjoyed myself but also felt a little awkward.

I would give myself a 90 percent for carrying out the plan. I did bring the wine and said thank you for inviting me. I talked to most of the people at the party.

Overall: Based on my experience, I have to say that my original prediction did not come true, and I can have a good time even if I don't know anyone where I am going. I can have conversations with people I don't know.

An experiment such as this helps you review your original beliefs. Before going to the party, you believed you weren't very interesting, and no one would find talking to you enjoyable. Now, you can reevaluate that belief. Your experiment disproved it. Although you might not be ready to believe that you are always going to enjoy parties when you don't know anyone, you accept it can sometimes happen. Your new belief might be…

I can sometimes enjoy parties even if I don't know anyone.

There are two types of goals: measuring success and measuring steps, called *intentional goals*. It is essential to focus on both. For example, if you want to lose 10 pounds, this is your overall or success goal. The steps you need to take, such as changing your diet and exercise habits, are your intentions. If you measure success at the intention level on a scale of 0 to 100 percent, it is easier to see where you can improve, and you are less likely to give up.

## Comparing Behaviors

You can also use planned experiments to test behaviors. Suppose you want to improve how you approach arguments with your partner. Your overall goal is to resolve the disagreement and develop a healthier relationship. You want to know what types of behaviors you could use to help reach this goal. To start, list several behaviors, or intention goals. For example:

- Agree to disagree. Because we both have opinions, it is impossible to agree on everything. If needed, look for compromises; if not, let it go, and accept we have different ideas.

- Acknowledge my partner's side of the argument without becoming defensive and critical. Use the sentence, "I understand you are upset because (fill in partner's reasons)" to let her know I heard what she said.
- Give each person a few minutes to cool down and then talk without interrupting each other.

Now, try out different behaviors to determine which works best for you. Keep a report card and use the same rating system, giving each action a score from 0 to 100 percent for how well you executed it and rate how much it contributed successfully to the outcome goal of resolving the fight.

**Report Card:**

Acknowledge the other person's side of the argument by saying, "I understand you are upset because…" without getting defensive and critical.

How well I did this: 80%.

How effective it was: 90%.

Notes: This was easier than I expected. Having a specific response gives me some control. This strategy opened the door to the other person and showed empathy for my side.

Give each of you a few minutes to cool down and then talking without interrupting each other.

How well I did this: 40%.

How effective it was: 90%.

Notes: This strategy was incredibly hard to pull off, but when I did, it helped.

A self-rated report card reviews the behaviors you used and how much each contributed to the outcome. As you continue to record and grade your actions, look back to determine which reaction gave you the most desirable outcome. In this example, resolving the argument and feeling more satisfied in the relationship. After you review your different approaches, you can conclude…

"Overall, during disagreements, using a statement to acknowledge his feelings and perspective works best. This approach ultimately leads to him wanting to know how I feel as well. We both end up feeling heard."

A behavior experiment also helps develop a level of comfort for a task you find difficult. Suppose you become anxious when you need to take an escalator. You want to lower your level of anxiety. Start by creating small steps, each one bringing you closer to being comfortable riding one.

Your actions and goals might be…

| Actions | Goal |
| --- | --- |
| Go to a building that has an escalator and watch people riding up and down. | Don't panic; if necessary, have a friend with me. |
| Pay attention to what causes the anxiousness. | Watch as one person walks to the escalator, gets on, and rides it to the floor above. Pay attention to which steps make you most anxious. Is it when the person stepped onto the escalator? Is it when the person rode up or stepped off? |
| Use the escalator with a friend. | Be able to ride the escalator with support. |
| Use the escalator alone. | Lowered feelings of anxiousness. |

Use the same report card system to chart your progress. Rate each action and each goal on a scale from 0 to 100 percent. Don't move to the next step until you have completed the task by at least 80 percent and the target by at least 90 percent.

# Feedback

Another type of behavioral experiment includes surveys and feedback. These work best with formal settings, such as work or school. In less-formal situations, informal feedback is more appropriate.

## Formal Surveys

Suppose you believe you are judged as inept any time you make a mistake at work. You hint to coworkers or your boss for feedback on your performance, but you aren't getting the right information. When you receive positive comments, you don't believe them. You still feel they judged you for any mistake. You can create a survey to test this negative thought process while gathering valuable information on your performance.

You might include questions such as the following:

- How would you rate my overall performance in the last 6 months?
- Was there a time in the last 6 months when you thought I was not doing enough? What precisely could I have done differently?
- What do you consider my areas of strength?
- What areas of my performance do you think need improvement?

Once you decide on a few questions, ask your boss to answer them. If there are other essential team members, ask them to complete it as well. The responses give you specific information to prove or disprove that your boss and coworkers are negatively judging you at work.

Sometimes, your original prediction is correct. For example, suppose your initial belief is, "My boss doesn't want to hear my ideas." Your experiment could prove this right. Think about whether the results say something about you or your boss. Is your boss not receptive or is it your delivery? While you might not like the results, you can now decide what is best for your life.

## Informal Surveys

In many situations, highly structured surveys are not appropriate. In these cases, informal ones work better. Use these with friends, significant others, and family.

*Situation:* I am having trouble finding a job.

*Problem:* I have gone on interviews I thought went well but have not had any job offers.

*Beliefs:* I am not good at interviewing. I won't ever get a job.

*Challenges to problematic thinking:* Overgeneralization. What part of the interview process needs improvement?

In this situation, think about people you know who are in a position to give you helpful information, for example, people who have hired employees. Reach out, explain your concerns, and ask for feedback on your interview skills. Discuss what you are wearing to interviews, how you present yourself, and what questions you ask. Let them know you want constructive feedback, such as suggestions on what to change and ideas on how to make those changes. Let them know this is not a pep rally, nor is it an opportunity to tear you down. Keep the conversation focused on specific topics. Let your friends know they can be honest and that you appreciate their feedback.

Write down everything they say and try not to react defensively. Initially, you might not want to hear the information, but after you've had time to reflect on the feedback, you can refer to your notes and make the appropriate changes.

Recognize that although you are not perfect and your friends' feedback is not the letter of the law, you now know some areas where you can improve and some things you did right.

## Observation

There might be times when you can't directly measure the results of your prediction by planning an experiment or taking a survey. At those times, observation works. Suppose you recently started a new job. To interact with your colleagues, you followed several on Instagram and invited them to follow you. You like or write comments on their posts and notice when they do the same for yours. But one person hasn't accepted your invitation even though she has an Instagram account. You take this to mean she doesn't like you and is not interested in becoming friends.

You decide to test your theory and determine if it's correct. First, come up with a few possible reasons for your coworker's behavior:

- She does not like me.
- She doesn't use social media often.
- She limits her interactions to people she knows well.

Because you can't determine what she is thinking and believe it is inappropriate to ask directly, you decide to observe her behavior on the site. You look at the posts that are not private and comment when appropriate. You check your other coworkers' posts and scan the comments and likes to see if she interacts with anyone. You scan comments on others' posts and check who has liked the posts. You notice that she is only following a few other coworkers and rarely comments or interacts with posts.

Your original theory has been proven incorrect. It isn't that your colleague doesn't like you; she is only minimally active on Instagram. The assumption that she doesn't use social media often is more likely than it is a personal affront to you.

Observations help when trying to decide which theory best fits the situation. This type of experiment enables you to create alternative views and opens you up to the possibility there is more than one explanation. Your observations should support or disprove your original hypothesis.

Each type of reality testing—formal, informal, or observation—has benefits. You need to decide which type is practical for the situation and which gives you the feedback you need to make positive changes in your thinking. No matter which model you choose, three key components help you create successful experiments.

*Expectations:* Establish clear expectations for what you want to achieve. Do this by breaking the overall goal into steps, the more specific, the better.

*Feedback:* Feedback is necessary. Use the 0 to 100 percent self-report card, and ask for input from others. Avoid becoming defensive because that leads to others not wanting to be honest.

*Reward:* Reward yourself for completing each step and moving closer to your overall goal; for example, use a star system for each level. When you achieve 10 stars, give yourself a tangible reward.

When reviewing results from reality testing, be sure to use your ABCDE chart to help you avoid reinforcing old beliefs.

# Your Turn: Testing Your Predictions

*The form accompanying this exercise is in Appendix C.*

Use the ABCDE log you created in previous exercises.

**A:** What is the situation or problem?

**B:** What are your negative beliefs about the situation?

**C:** What do you assume will happen?

**D:** What are your problematic thought processes, and how can you challenge them?

**E:** Which type of reality test would best fit this situation? What action plan can you use to prove or disprove your theory? What action plan can you use to achieve your overall goal?

Determine a reward for each action and for achieving your overall goal.

Remember, feedback does not necessarily need to be from other people. Rating your goals with the 0 to 100 percent scale is also feedback. Keep a notebook of your reality tests and refer to the results when a similar situation comes up.

In CBT, you look for negative thought processes and replace them with a positive perspective. Reality testing helps you prove or disprove thoughts and decide whether your thinking is helpful or harmful. Think of it as a scientist looking for evidence to back up his theory. You can also use it to choose what behavior would be best in a situation or to request feedback on your actions and thinking patterns.

# PART 3

# CBT for Personal Growth

Your thoughts have an effect on every part of your life. They reflect how you feel about yourself, how you interact with others, and how you handle stressful situations. When you use negative thoughts and words to describe yourself, it creates negativity in all these areas. CBT helps you reframe and restructure your thoughts into more positive views. With practice and commitment, these changes become lasting and permanent, improving your sense of well-being.

In this part, we discuss areas of personal growth, such as boosting self-esteem, improving communication, letting go of perfectionism, and building relationships. Finally, we talk about learning to manage the stress in your life by giving you step-by-step ways to break problems down and solve them one at a time. As you focus on one area, you might notice other parts of your life improving as well.

# CHAPTER 11
# Increasing Your Self-Esteem

Do you like yourself? Are you happy with who you are? Self-esteem reflects how you think about yourself. If you are like many people, you don't love yourself all the time. It is possible, however, to choose how you feel about yourself. In this chapter, we talk about what self-esteem is, identify obstacles to creating a healthy self-image, and discover ways to improve self-esteem and learn self-acceptance.

## What Do We Mean by Self-Esteem?

Self-esteem refers to your opinion of your overall value and self-worth. If you use negative words to describe yourself, such as failure, loser, idiot, stupid, or lazy, you probably have low self-esteem. You might use external factors to measure your self-worth, such as your appearance, job, or relationships. But self-worth is not just about what you offer others; you have value as a person.

You might think of low self-esteem as something to improve, or you might believe you need to develop high self-esteem. After all, high is the opposite of low. But both low and high self-esteem are products of self-judgment. The opposite of low self-esteem is self-acceptance—accepting who you are and understanding that while you are fallible, you are a complex human being with strengths and weaknesses.

## Self-Acceptance

Self-acceptance is unconditional. It recognizes your weaknesses, faults, and limitations and accepts that these do not define who you are or your self-worth. Self-acceptance means liking yourself—your whole self. It is viewing weaknesses as areas to improve rather than as failures.

Your level of self-acceptance often determines how happy you are in life. In his book, *Happiness Now!*, author Robert Holden explains that you allow yourself to experience happiness only to the degree that you believe you are worthy of it. If you don't accept yourself, you don't think you deserve to be happy; if you do, you allow yourself to enjoy life.

Your level of self-acceptance can vary in different areas of your life. For example, at work, you could exhibit confidence and are assured you mastered the duties of your job; when you make a mistake, you accept responsibility and shift into problem-solving mode. Your overall belief is that you are competent and capable. However, you might be unsure of yourself in personal relationships. You feel guilty for not spending enough time with your family and berate yourself for not showing enough consideration. Your confidence level at work is high, but it drops when you arrive home.

Self-acceptance allows you to take responsibility for your actions without becoming defensive. You see negative feedback as critique, not criticism. You are open to growth and learning.

A cynical view of yourself is limiting. If you think, "I am a failure," you give up trying because you believe it doesn't matter how much you try because you will fail. Negative thinking can take away the motivation to change and improve. With self-acceptance, you see yourself objectively and take responsibility for limitations. For example, if you are consistently late for work, you might think, "I am late too often. Let me figure out the reasons why and decide what to do to prevent this in the future."

## Obstacles to Self-Acceptance

There are two main components to developing self-acceptance:

- Recognizing strengths and successes.
- Recognizing and being comfortable with shortcomings and mistakes.

Knowing your strengths sounds easier than it is. The problematic thought processes explained in Chapter 2, such as focusing on the negative and minimizing achievements, interfere with seeing positive traits. Negative thinking patterns are obstacles to self-acceptance.

### Equating Acceptance with Giving Up

One myth about self-acceptance is that once you accept a fault, you resign yourself to always having it. You believe it is a permanent trait, and you agree it is part of you. But self-acceptance doesn't work that way. It doesn't mean giving up or giving in. It means accepting limitations and finding ways to improve. For example, suppose you have test anxiety. When you were in school, you struggled. You studied and knew the work, but when it came time to take a test, you froze.

Your grades suffered. Now as an adult, you are considering taking classes to further your career, but your mind keeps going back to your previous school experience, and you hesitate. You can choose to give up on the idea of going back to school, or you can accept if you reach out for help, there are ways to help you combat test anxiety. The second option recognizes your limitations and looks for strategies to improve.

## Measuring Your Worth on External Factors

You could equate your self-worth with external factors, such as your job, financial status, attractiveness, or love life. But these situations are often temporary and can change without warning, causing your view of your self-worth to plummet. You should base self-worth on who you are, not what you do for a living, whether you have money in the bank, or whether you are in a relationship. Basing it on external factors means it fluctuates when those factors change.

## Overgeneralizing

Overgeneralizing is another problematic thought process that contributes to low self-esteem. When you make one mistake, you globalize it and believe you are a failure. When one situation goes wrong, you assume you are doomed and everything will go wrong. You fail to see occurrences as single incidents; instead, you lump them together, even when they are unrelated.

## Maintaining an Outdated Self-Image

Life is ever changing. We aren't the same people we were 5 or 10 years ago. Since then, experience has taught us lessons, and our perspectives on life have probably changed. But many people don't adjust their self-images. They continue to see themselves as they were. Suppose you weren't popular in high school. Years later, you have a circle of friends and enjoy their company, as they do yours. Even so, you still see yourself as alone and unpopular. You haven't updated your self-image to reflect today's reality.

## Basing Self-Worth on One Aspect

Human beings are complicated, with many aspects of personality and varied talents and abilities. Some people look at just one trait and spin it as unfavorable. Suppose you are artistic. You regularly receive compliments on your work, but you don't enjoy sports and have never been good at them. In your mind, your nonathleticism tops your list of traits rather than your artistic abilities.

# Your Turn: Self-Assessment

*The form accompanying this exercise is in Appendix C.*

For each of the following categories, write down a few short statements that describe you. Don't think too hard. Write down thoughts that immediately come to mind.

- Physical appearance
- Interpersonal skills
- Problem-solving
- Creativity
- Sexuality
- Productivity at work or school
- Personal productivity
- How others see you

Once you are done, look at the list and highlight every negative word. Use a different color to highlight the positive words. Use the descriptions of problematic thought processes in Chapter 2 to find the ones you use in your self-descriptions and then write positive thoughts to replace each negative one. Read your new list aloud each day.

# Steps to Improving Self-Esteem

It is impossible to rid yourself of shortcomings. The idea of self-acceptance isn't to make yourself perfect; it is to accept yourself, faults and all. It is admitting you are a unique individual and knowing you have something to offer other people. Recognizing shortcomings doesn't make you less of a person or less valuable to others. People who practice self-acceptance focus on growth and improvement; people with low self-esteem focus on not making mistakes.

## Monitor and Adjust Your Self-Talk

The self-assessment you completed in the previous exercise identified your negative self-perceptions. Listening to your negative self-talk and the negative messages you send yourself is the first step to improving your self-esteem. Now, reword those messages as positive, relevant descriptions.

Under *Work*, suppose your characteristics include the following:

- Careless. I make a lot of mistakes.
- Lazy. I leave work earlier than my coworkers.

When reviewing problematic thinking processes, you realized you overgeneralize, label, ignore the positive, and think in black and white. You focused on what you felt was wrong instead of finding positive traits. Your revised statements might be...

- I am usually conscientious about my work. There are times I feel overwhelmed.
- I am usually the first person here in the morning, and I often work through lunch. I am hardworking.

As you go through your day, notice when you repeat one of your negative statements in your mind. Each time you do, you reinforce it. Focus on catching yourself and repeating the revised description.

When altering negative self-talk, use accurate and logical language. Your mind resists false statements. For example, don't use "I am the most conscientious worker." Create a positive, accurate statement, such as, "I am a hard worker."

## Review Your Expectations

Your self-esteem takes a hit when you set a goal or create expectations for a situation and then fall short or when the reality is much different than you imagined. You might feel you failed, but maybe your expectations were unrealistic. Suppose you start a new job and think, "I will learn this job in my first week." You have given yourself an unrealistic goal because most jobs take more than 1 week to learn. With your goal, when Friday afternoon comes and you don't know everything, you feel disappointed. You think you are a failure, stupid, and unqualified because you didn't live up to your self-imposed expectations. It could be helpful to review SMART goal setting in Chapter 5, and decide whether your expectations are realistic.

Try to look at situations with self-efficacy, which means you can handle a situation. It doesn't necessarily mean you know what you are doing but that you have the resources and capabilities to figure things out.

## Don't Compare Yourself to Others

Self-esteem suffers when you compare yourself to others. Comparisons end with you being better or worse than the other person, usually worse. Your neighbor bought a new car, and you feel inadequate about your vehicle. Your friend bought a new house, and it is bigger and more modern than yours. Your sister got a new job, and it pays more than yours. When you compare yourself to someone else, you usually believe you are inferior. Focus instead on your own goals. Other people's achievements and possessions have nothing to do with you. Be happy for them and proud of your accomplishments.

## Add Self-Esteem Activities

Your beliefs about yourself could stop you from trying new things or participating in activities. You might use self-talk to make excuses for not doing something, even if you would enjoy it. For example, you consider joining a hiking group, but you tell yourself you aren't good at hiking. Instead of giving it a try and learning something new, you stop yourself before giving yourself a chance to improve.

Think about something you haven't done yet—something you daydreamed about it but haven't dared try. Set a goal and create the steps needed to get to the desired outcome. If it is the hiking group, your plan might be to go on one hike or to look for a beginner's group. Look for activities that allow you to feel good about yourself.

# Your Turn: Create Mini Action Plans

Keep track of thoughts about yourself and create small actions to help counter negative thoughts or images. Remember to be specific, flexible, and positive.

Set a timer for 5 minutes and write five positive things about yourself in the following categories:

- Strengths
- Achievements
- Activities you enjoy
- What you admire about yourself
- What makes you feel good about yourself

Don't worry about grammar or spelling. Simply focus on the positives in your life.

## Accepting Bad Behavior

Learning to change your thought process, while never simple, might seem impossible if you feel guilt and shame about something that occurred in your past. Suppose you…

- Stole money from your employer.
- Shoplifted.
- Had an affair.
- Lost your temper and hurt someone.
- Feel guilty about anything you have done.

You might believe you are a terrible person. Every time you tell yourself something good, you remind yourself of your misdeed. Your guilt and shame override any positive statement.

Self-acceptance means accepting yourself, flaws and all. It means you acknowledge you are fallible and imperfect. You make mistakes, but your mistakes don't define you. At the same time, take responsibility for your error, own up to it, and if necessary, make restitution or apologize. Acknowledge the pain you caused someone and accept the consequences of your action. Avoiding it increases your guilt. Accept your apology for what it is. You cannot make someone forgive you; you can only control forgiving yourself.

When you accept and own up to a mistake, you acknowledge it does not define you, make you worthless, or make you a terrible person. It makes you a person who made a mistake.

It isn't possible to change the past, but you can change how you perceive and respond to it (or the memory of it). Look objectively at the event that causes guilt. Reframe the memory to include what you learned from the incident and how it helped you grow. Think about what you can learn from this mistake. What can you do to make sure it doesn't happen again?

It is difficult to come to terms with a mistake, especially if others were hurt emotionally or physically, but forgiveness is possible. Continue focusing on your self-talk and monitor it for negative thought patterns. Continue to work on adopting a more helpful way of thinking.

Self-acceptance is hard. It means you need to like yourself—faults and all. How you talk to yourself can feed into a negative view of yourself, or it could raise your self-esteem. Listen to your inner narration and adjust to a more positive outlook if necessary. Watch for thoughts comparing yourself to others. Another downfall when trying to increase self-esteem is equating bad behavior with being a terrible person. Instead, accept you can be a good person who has made a mistake.

# CHAPTER 12
# Overcoming Perfectionism

Striving for excellence is an admirable trait, but there is a fine line between striving for excellence and the need to be perfect. In this chapter, you learn what perfectionism is, learn how perfectionism negatively affects your life, and learn strategies to lessen your expectations while still putting your best self forward.

## Defining Perfectionism

Perfectionism includes self-imposed, extremely high standards. A perfectionist continually works to attain these standards, even when it interferes with their life or relationships. When you set incredibly high standards for yourself, you often feel like nothing is good enough. Trying to achieve perfection frequently causes frustration, anxiety, and depression.

Imagine you are completing a report for work. You spend several hours compiling the information. You want to make sure it is correct and spend hours double-and triple-checking the research for accuracy. Then you ask two coworkers to check your work. When you receive it back, you recheck it again. A 1 day report took 3 days because you needed to check the job repeatedly. Your boss is upset that you handed in the report late. Although your work might have been perfect, it didn't matter because you missed your deadline.

You could be a perfectionist in everything you do, or you might have high standards in some areas of your life. For example, suppose you play baseball. You are passionate about the sport and want to win every game. You spend hours practicing hitting and throwing the ball. You expect your teammates to do the same and are annoyed when they don't even show up for practice. You blame yourself if your team loses, believing if you had hit the ball farther or ran a little faster, you would have won. You spend even more time practicing after a loss. Because of the time you spend on baseball, your work and relationships suffer—all your goals center on being a perfect baseball player.

Perfectionism usually comes at a cost. The following are some of the negative ways perfectionism affects your life:

- You lack free time.
- You neglect some areas of your life.
- Achievements feel empty or do not satisfy you.
- You blame yourself when things don't go right or the way you want them done.
- You blame others when things aren't done "the right way" or your way.
- You don't believe others can do the job as well as you.
- You waste time doing tasks several times to make sure they are done correctly.
- You feel judged if things are not perfect.
- You always worry about not being good enough.
- You procrastinate or avoid doing things because you don't think you will do them correctly.

Perfectionism can have both negative and positive effects on health. When you use perfectionism to motivate you to succeed, it has a positive effect on health. However, when you believe others are judging you as perfect or not perfect, there is an adverse effect, and it results in a higher risk of developing physical illnesses.

It is essential to set goals and to have high standards. But if your quest for excellence interferes with other parts of your life or causes frustration and anxiety, you need to learn ways to scale back your expectations.

## Your Turn: Are You a Perfectionist?

Read the following statements and think about if you agree. Respond with *always*, *frequently*, *rarely*, or *never*.

1. Making mistakes causes problems.
2. I spend so much time making sure I complete tasks correctly that I often don't have time to finish the rest of my work or do other things.
3. I feel it is essential to do things right the first time.
4. I avoid doing tasks I don't think I can do perfectly.

5. I believe other people think badly of me if I do not do jobs right.

6. I need to do everything well, even those things that I know I do not do well.

7. When I do accomplish something, I don't think it is enough. I always think there is something more I could have done.

If you responded "always" or "frequently" to most of the statements, chances are that perfectionism causes problems for you.

# Perfectionist Thought Patterns

Problematic thought patterns are inaccurate ways of interpreting the world around you; check Chapter 2 for common ones. Those often seen in perfectionism include the ones shown in the following sections.

## Black-and-White Thinking

Everything is either good or bad. You don't see any gray area. Therefore, if a situation is not perfect, it is unacceptable. Examples of this type of thinking pattern in perfectionism include the following:

- If it isn't perfect, it is a failure.
- If I can't do it correctly, I might as well not try at all.
- I am either a loser or a winner; I'm either successful or a failure.

## Catastrophizing

Every problem ends in disaster. You believe any mistake is unacceptable, no matter how small. Examples of this type of thinking in perfectionism include the following:

- If I make a mistake, everyone will think I am stupid.
- I can't handle the humiliation of making a mistake.

Do something bad. Go ahead, try something new, and intentionally fail at it. Learn from your mistake. You should learn two things: one, how to do it better, and two, nothing happened. You didn't die, and you didn't stop breathing, everyone didn't stand in a circle around you, pointing and laughing. Life went on. Go on, go out, and do something badly.

## Personalization and Blame

Everything that goes wrong is your fault, or you blame others because they didn't live up to your high standards. You say things like…

- We would have won the baseball game if I had practiced more during the week.
- We would have won the baseball game if the other players took it seriously and showed up for practice.
- Why can't my employees just listen to me and do things correctly?
- I am better off doing everything myself; others are just lazy and stupid.

## "Should" and "Must"

Everyone needs to live up to your high standards, and you are frustrated and angry when they don't. You feel guilty if you do not do everything exactly right. This type of thinking may lead to statements such as…

- Mistakes are bad; I should never make a mistake.
- I must always make sure my work is perfect before I hand it in.
- Everyone should work as hard as I do. I work over the weekends; why shouldn't they?

## Mind Reading

You assume other people follow the same rules as you do and feel angry when they live by different rules. You lack empathy and consideration for how others think.

- My coworkers never check emails in the evening or over the weekend. What is wrong with them?
- My friend didn't invite my partner to join in; I would never do such a thing. She is rude and inconsiderate.

# Adding Flexibility to Your Life

We all have specific "rules" that guide how we live. Community-based rules include, "It is important to be kind to others," or "Lying is wrong." You follow these rules most of the time but also understand that they are flexible. You might not be kind to people every moment of every day, yet you still consider yourself a kind person. Rules such as these are essential and are usually helpful in your life. They become unhelpful when rigid or inflexible; for example, you believe you are a failure when you make a mistake.

## Revising Rigid Rules

Think about the expectations you set for yourself and others. Do you have high expectations for yourself? Do you believe others should live up to your expectations? Do you get hurt, angry, anxious, or disappointed when things don't go your way? Is it difficult for you to revise goals and expectations when they seem unreasonable or unattainable? If you have a hard time doing so or find you are judging others for not living up to your standards, it would be helpful for you to revise your life rules.

When trying to be more flexible or to see something from a different perspective, try changing your physical environment. Go for a walk, sit in a different chair, or move to a separate room. Sometimes, changing your visual perspective helps you think differently.

Consider the following examples of rigid rules and how you can reword them to incorporate flexibility.

*Rigid rule:* Others should not ask personal questions until they get to know me better.

*Flexible rule:* Sometimes, people ask personal questions to get to know me. I have the right to decline to answer if it makes me uncomfortable.

*Rigid rule:* Everyone should work as hard as I do.

*Flexible rule:* It is my choice to work this hard. Others can make their own decisions.

*Rigid rule:* I cannot make a mistake, or I will look foolish.

*Flexible rule:* Everyone makes mistakes. It is okay if I make a mistake.

*Rigid rule:* I must do everything entirely and perfectly before letting someone else see it.

*Flexible rule:* It is okay to show someone a draft or a work in progress.

When you find yourself feeling disappointed in your behavior or the behavior of others, think about your expectation. Is it rigid or flexible? Write down your rule and then create a more flexible version of the statement. The ABCD charts you completed in previous chapters can help you discover your rigid rules and modify your expectations and thoughts.

## Perfectionist Behavior Checklist

Perfectionism shows up in your behaviors, leaving you feeling overwhelmed. Review the following statements and check off those relevant to your life:

- ❏ Indecisive; you are unable to decide because you are afraid of making the wrong decision.
- ❏ Overly organized; you write and rewrite lists, you believe everything has its place, and you feel uncomfortable when or if things are out of order.

- ❏ You must have your workspace organized before you can start work.
- ❏ You check over your work several times to make sure it is correct.
- ❏ You ask others to check your work to make sure it is acceptable.
- ❏ You avoid tasks you think you can't complete perfectly.
- ❏ You correct other people when they make a small mistake, such as mispronounce a word or say something incorrectly.
- ❏ You comment when you think someone says something politically incorrect and try to persuade them into thinking like you.
- ❏ You clean your bathroom and kitchen with antiseptic cleansers every day to make sure there aren't any germs.
- ❏ When giving instructions, you fill in every possible detail.
- ❏ You never throw away paperwork, such as bank statements and tax returns, just in case you need the information.
- ❏ You do all the work yourself, at home and work, because you don't trust anyone else to do it correctly.
- ❏ You redo another person's work because "it's just not good enough."
- ❏ You demand others do things your way.

These are some examples of perfectionist behaviors; you might notice others in your life. When you find yourself behaving in these ways, stop and ask yourself if you are doing so because you are trying to meet your incredibly high standards. If so, try to modify your behaviors to reflect more flexible thinking.

## Introduce Shades of Grey into Your Life

Usually, problematic thinking that leads to perfectionism contains absolutes. You think that something must be done a certain way or it is wrong; you believe that if you don't do something perfectly, it isn't worth doing. Changing perfectionism doesn't mean giving up on your standards; it means introducing shades of gray into your life.

You might notice that perfectionism does not show up in every area of your life, and it might not interfere with some areas as much as with others. To start reducing perfectionist tendencies, consider where your quest for excellence is causing the most problems. For example,

- Do you have trouble getting things at work accomplished because you want everything to be perfect?
- Is your relationship in trouble because you expect your partner to do everything your way?

- Do you exercise or diet constantly because you need to have a perfect body?
- Do you neglect certain parts of your life because you spend too much time on others? What are those areas?

Once you decide where you want to start, consider which high standards are the most important to you. Remember, the goal is not to settle but to limit your high ideals to things that matter.

## Your Turn: Shades of Gray

Make a list of your expectations for a given task. Once you meet those standards, stop working on the task to prevent you from wasting time seeking the "best" or "most perfect thing." For example, suppose you are shopping for a pair of running shoes. Make a list of three features you want in your new shoes. You might want…

- Proper fit
- Good for cross-training
- Cost no more than $60

Keep your list with you when you shop. Once you find a pair of shoes that fit your criteria, buy them and end your shopping trip. Don't visit more stores to see if you can find something better. You know you have a product that meets your criteria. You are not settling; you are preventing yourself from wasting time trying to find the "perfect shoe."

Limiting your choices requires you to choose between what is available instead of endlessly searching for the perfect choice. For example, if you agonize each morning trying to find the ideal outfit to wear to work, try taking out several outfits the evening before. In the morning, choose from one of those outfits rather than going through all your clothes.

## Cost-Benefit Analysis

At first, lessening your expectations feels uncomfortable. You fight the urge to continue to live up to your high standards. You might find it helpful to list the negative consequences of one high standard you typically use. For the preceding example, your list might include the following:

- Spent my entire day going to shoe stores
- Wasted gas driving around
- Spent extra money buying coffee and lunch to keep my energy up
- Missed out on getting together with friends because of my need to find the perfect shoe
- Ended up going over my budget

Reminding yourself of the negative consequences of your perfectionism keeps you motivated to change. Reward yourself, even if it is a virtual pat on the back, each time you follow your new standard. Remember, everyone makes mistakes, so if you slip and go to one other shoe store, don't judge yourself; just review your goals and commitment to change and start again.

# Procrastination and Perfectionism

If you are a perfectionist, you might avoid doing things that you can't do perfectly. You prefer not to do something rather than fail. Procrastination, or avoidance, is a frequent partner to perfectionism.

Imagine you have a report to complete for work. You don't have a specific deadline, but you know your boss is waiting for it. Even so, you keep putting off starting. You want it to be perfect; anything less is a failure. When you find yourself avoiding a task, ask yourself these questions:

- Am I striving for excellence or demanding perfection?
- Is the result going to matter in my life next month, next year, or 5 years from now?
- Do I want to do well because this is something that matters to me or because I want others to think well of me?
- What is the worst thing that could happen if it is not perfect? How am I going to manage that?

Use the following strategies to help you deal with procrastination:

*Create a definite beginning to your project.* Select an exact time to start instead of waiting until you "feel like doing something."

*Set a specific ending time.* Don't allow yourself to review or redo tasks to make them better. End at the time you set.

*Use a timer.* Give yourself a specific amount of time to work on a task and set a timer to go off 5 minutes before to warn you time is almost up. Then, reset it to go off at the ending time. When the second timer rings, stop working.

*Break tasks into precise measurable chunks.* For example, "read pages 20-40." Then schedule your time based on how much you need to do only this.

These strategies might feel uncomfortable at first. You might worry about the quality of your work. When you were in school, the quality was crucial. Mistakes resulted in poor grades. But when you enter the working world, this changes. Productivity and meeting deadlines are valued. Companies usually do not base promotions and raises on flawless work; employees who can get the job done on time are more apt to receive a raise. With practice, you gain confidence in your abilities and find it easier to resist triple- or quadruple-checking your work.

# Your Turn: Taking One Step at a Time

*The form accompanying this exercise is in Appendix C.*

When working toward a goal, it helps to break it into steps. The stepladder approach outlined in Chapter 5 works well for overcoming perfectionism. Start with the top and bottom rungs of the ladder. On the bottom rung, list the perfectionism behavior you want to change. On the top rung, write down your goal—how you want your action to look. Create intermediate goals on each rung. Suppose you check your work three times and have a coworker check it once before handing it in. Your ladder may look like this:

> Top rung: Check work once, and hand it in.
>
> Third rung: Check work twice, and hand it in.
>
> Second rung: Check work twice, and have a coworker check it.
>
> Bottom rung: Check work three times, and have a coworker check it.

Rather than trying to reach your goal in one step, you have a plan of action. Start at the bottom rung and work your way up. Depending on your goal, your ladder could have more or fewer rungs. Remember, when you first begin, you might feel some anxiety. Hang in there and resist the urge to resort to your perfectionism behaviors. If you do give in, it could be even more challenging next time.

Perfectionism is the result of self-imposed standards. You believe everything must live up to your definition of excellence. Anything less is a failure. Living with perfectionism could cost you in failed relationships, poor performance at work because of missed deadlines, and frustration. Avoidance of a task, or procrastination, is often a result of perfectionism because you avoid some tasks due to your fear of failure. Creating more realistic expectations and limiting your choices helps manage perfectionism.

# CHAPTER 13
# Improving Your Relationships

Relationships bring joy to your life. It is wonderful to know there is someone by your side to share the great moments and offer support during the not-so-good ones. But when there are problems, these same relationships cause pain, anxiety, and stress. This chapter identifies some of the common issues that occur in a relationship and provides strategies for dealing with them. Although we focus on the relationship between partners, the concepts and skills are helpful in any relationship.

## Who Is to Blame?

Your relationship isn't working, or maybe you hit a bumpy patch. You love your partner but feel neglected, misunderstood, disrespected, or criticized. You aren't sure what went wrong, but lately, you argue more than talk. When you attempt to resolve differences, you end up fighting or you ignore each other.

You might think…

- We are not communicating at all. Why bother trying?
- My partner never listens to me. He doesn't care about my opinion. This marriage is hopeless.
- My partner wants everything done her way. I am sick of it.
- My partner turns down my advances all the time. I am not loved or attractive.
- Get off my back. My partner always tells me I am wrong.

No matter what the issues are, chances are you blame your partner for many problems in your relationship. You think if you could fix them, everything would be okay. But improving a relationship isn't about fixing the other person. Both people are responsible for the health of the relationship, and both people are responsible when things aren't working. It is best when both people work together to solve problems within a relationship. However, when you focus on what you can do to improve the relationship, things could change for the better.

Who is to blame? Both of you. The problems in a relationship are usually not the fault of one person. (Abuse is an exception to this rule. If your partner is physically, emotionally, or financially abusing you, it is not your fault, and you should reach out for help.)

People frequently use blame to protect their self-esteem. It is easier to make someone else wrong than it is to accept responsibility. Most people, even those who blame their spouse for marriage problems, understand that they must take at least partial responsibility for the issues. This chapter outlines changes you can make in yourself to change your perspective, actions, and reactions. Hopefully by doing so, you can improve your relationship.

## Choose Your Reaction

Your significant other gives you negative feedback. Your immediate reaction might be "He is always critical of me. He makes me so angry." Your shoulders tense up, and you are ready to react by defending yourself and pointing out his faults in retaliation. You keep going over his words in your mind. Your anger builds, and you blame him for your feelings. After all, you weren't mad before he criticized you.

In reality, no one creates your feelings; you are solely responsible for your emotions. You might reject the notion that you chose to be angry, but you always pick how to react to a situation. Sometimes, you respond quickly and don't stop to analyze why. You believe your first reaction, anger, and it colors further interactions. CBT tells you to slow down, look at your underlying thoughts, and address the inaccuracies in those instead of lashing out.

We usually react to problems in one of two ways: emotionally or practically. Anger, happiness, excitement, and sadness are all emotional reactions. Practical reactions include "This is a problem; what should I do next?" Our feelings frequently overrule practicality and can cover up an underlying negative thought pattern. In the previous example, your reaction might mask thoughts such as, "I am not good enough," "I am not important," or "I need to be perfect." This anger could be the result of fear that your underlying thoughts are real. For example, when your spouse corrects, criticizes, or offers advice, your emotional reaction might mask the idea that "If he is right, then it is true that I am not good enough." Your response, not his, reinforced your negative thought patterns.

Think back (or keep track over the next few weeks) to your adverse reactions in your relationship. Ask yourself what you are feeling and why. See if there is a pattern and try to discern what thought processes you follow most often. Come up with coping statements to address these issues. Keep in mind that you choose how you react.

## Making Demands

You grew up with an image in your mind of the ideal relationship. For years, you honed this image, and you expect your relationship to mirror it. You created certain expectations in your mind, including how you expect your significant other to act in a variety of situations. Early in the relationship, you might follow "love is blind" and ignore it when she doesn't meet those expectations. Sooner or later, though, you expect her to fall in line with your image. You fill your relationships with "should" and "must" statements.

Dr. Aaron Beck, who is sometimes referred to as the "father of CBT," coined the term MUSTerbation to refer to emotional and cognitive demands placed on yourself, others, or a group of people. In addition to "should" and "must," MUSTerbation uses terms such as "need," or "have to." MUSTERbations are demands you put on yourself, others, or the circumstances, and they are frequently the source of conflict.

For example:

- I must be a perfect spouse.
- We should not fight.
- We should always be happy.
- I should always be first in her life.
- He should always want to spend time with me.

When you use "should" and "must" statements, you don't leave room for exceptions. If you believe that in happy marriages, spouses don't fight, any argument in your marriage must signal a serious problem. "Must" and "should" beliefs might be masked by your emotions. For example, you are telling your spouse about your day and realize she is distracted and has not been listening. You become angry. But the act of not listening is not what caused your distress; it is that she broke one of your rules: My spouse should always listen when I talk. You might also attach an emotional response to this demand, such as "If she doesn't listen, she doesn't love me."

Use an ABC chart to help identify underlying "should" or "must" demands.

| A: Activating Event | B: "Should" or "Must" Statement | C: Emotion |
|---|---|---|
| Spouse continued to watch television while I was talking. | He **should** listen to me when I am talking. | Angry |

Once you identify your "should" or "must" statement, create a healthier way to look at the situation. Make a conscious choice to turn your demand into a preference. "I would prefer that he gives me his undivided attention when I talk." Preferences allow for exceptions and can reduce or eliminate anger.

When disputing "should" and "must" statements, remember the following:

- Your partner is an individual with free will.
- Your partner has the right to make her own decisions.
- Your partner does not need to do what you want or agree with you all the time.
- When your partner does not follow your expectations, it does not mean he does not love you.

Some people find it helpful to turn their expectations into a question, such as "Why must she listen with undivided attention every time I speak?" While it might be unpleasant when your partner does not agree with you or meet your expectations, as an adult, you can handle the disappointment.

"Should" and "must" statements reflect inflexible or rigid thinking. When questioning these types of thoughts, ask yourself what you would tell a friend who was in your situation. For example, if a friend called and said his partner did not give her undivided attention, what would you say? You might tell him that if something is significant, he should ask if she can turn off the TV while they talk. Or you might suggest giving his partner a heads up, "I would prefer your undivided attention when we are talking." You might say, "This isn't a big deal. Haven't you ever been talking with someone and suddenly realized your mind wandered, and you don't know what they said." Use the same advice you would give your friend when restructuring your thoughts.

## Your Turn: Sharing Preferences

*The form accompanying this exercise is in Appendix C.*

Over the next week, use the ABC chart to note when you feel frustrated or disappointed in your relationship.

Use the information to determine your "should" and "must" expectations.

Rewrite each into a preference.

At the end of the week, cross out any preferences you think are unreasonable for your relationship.

Set up a time to talk with your partner about the preferences left on your list. You can start the conversation with "I have some ideas about how we should treat each other. I want to share these ideas with you and would like to hear your input."

Ask your partner to write down his preferences. When he shares his list, be sure not to interrupt or correct him until it is your turn to give feedback.

## Breaking the Cycle

Unmet expectations in your marriage might start a vicious cycle. For example, you are upset that your partner frequently works late, and your time together is limited. By the time he arrives home, your resentment has simmered for hours, and you are hurt and annoyed; sometimes, you ignore him to punish him for working late. Your partner doesn't like coming home because you are often angry. Whenever his boss asks someone to stay late, he volunteers. This cycle continues until you and your partner barely speak to one another.

While it is best to work through relationship problems together, with both partners involved in the solution, either partner can make changes and stop the cycle. By changing your perception, behavior, and reaction to the situation, you change the dynamics.

Let's look at the scenario again.

You are upset that your partner has been working late and is not home for dinner. You react by saying, "I miss having dinner together, and I miss you. I enjoy seeing you in the evenings. Let's plan for a special dinner this week. What night works best for you?" In this response, you let your partner know your feelings without making demands. He is more likely to be responsive to your request. You have broken the cycle of tense evenings.

When you and your partner are in a rut, try complimenting your partner. It is easy to focus on the negative elements of your partner and your relationship. Instead, tell your partner something you appreciate. If an argument is going in circles, take a break. When you come back to the topic, start by telling each other something you like about the other person to help break the cycle and remind you of why you are together.

# Communication Skills

Every relationship has a conflict at some point. It is not the problem but rather how you handle it, that leads to either a disagreement or solution. What you say is vital to effective communication, but your behavior—your nonverbal communication—says just as much as your words, if not more.

## Listening

Do you actively listen when others talk? Do you focus on what someone says, or do you start forming a response before she finishes? Many people believe they are listening and don't even realize that they are thinking about what to say next. Active listening means you hear the words spoken and understand the feelings behind the words.

The following are some guidelines for active listening:

- Maintain eye contact.
- Don't interrupt. If you feel a response is needed, nod, smile, or use another type of body language to indicate you are listening.
- Reflect what you heard. Reword and repeat vital information to let your partner know you are listening.
- Ask clarifying questions to make sure you understand what the other person is saying.
- Pay attention to your partner's body language and other nonverbal cues to get a better sense of his feelings.
- Monitor your body language. Show you are listening by leaning in, nodding, smiling, and making eye contact.

When listening, avoid offering advice unless the other person explicitly asks for it. When you listen, the other person feels worthy, appreciated, and respected. It helps prevent misunderstandings. You always learn more when you listen than when you talk.

Keep any criticism or judgments to yourself while your partner is talking. You want to foster an environment of open and honest communication, so even if you don't agree, keep your opinions to yourself while your partner is speaking. Try to understand their perspective.

## Speaking

There could be times when you think your partner is the one who needs to learn how to listen. You might feel frustrated or believe your spouse doesn't listen to you. How you approach a conversation is essential. The following are guidelines for being heard:

- Find the right time. Don't try to have a meaningful discussion when the television is on or when one of you is preoccupied with other issues. It might help to schedule a time, so both can prepare to have a discussion.
- Avoid attacking or cross-examining during your turn to talk.

- Keep your body language consistent with the message you are trying to deliver.
- Edit what you want to say. Stop if you begin rambling, going off topic, repeating yourself, or attacking the other person.
- Pause occasionally to allow your partner to ask questions. Ask for feedback to make it a two-way conversation.

Let your partner know your intentions before you begin the conversation. For example, you might want advice or to vent. You might want to collaborate to solve a problem. Each of these requires a different response. State in advance which response you want, so you aren't disappointed or frustrated. If you are asking for advice, however, be ready to accept it graciously. That doesn't mean you need to heed the recommendations, but don't be critical or harshly dismiss the advice.

## Nonverbal Communication

Your body language, or nonverbal communication, says a great deal about the feelings behind your words. Your partner unconsciously reads your body language. Sometimes, it reflects your words, but other times, it doesn't. For example, if you are annoyed but trying to hide that emotion, your body language probably gives you away. Becoming aware of your body language and the body language of your partner makes you a better communicator.

Nonverbal communication includes eye contact, gestures, tone of voice, muscle tension, facial expression, and body movements. The following tips will help you notice and use nonverbal cues to improve your communication.

*Notice when nonverbal cues don't match up with the words.* Maybe your partner's words indicate he isn't upset, but he has his arms crossed and is looking away from you. His nonverbal communication is sending a different message than his words. When this happens, ask questions to find out more. Unexpressed anger often turns into resentment.

*Use eye contact.* When you are unwilling to make eye contact, it gives the impression you are trying to hide something. Too much eye contact can seem confrontational. Be sure to make eye contact without trying to stare down your partner.

*Don't focus on one small gesture.* You can better understand the meaning behind nonverbal communication if you look at more than one movement or gesture. When a group of nonverbal cues reinforces an idea or an emotion, you are probably reading the signals correctly.

Touching or smiling can change the tone of adverse situations. If you and your partner had an argument and you are still upset and replaying the disagreement in your mind or are unable to let go, try holding hands, hugging, snuggling together, or giving a simple smile or touch. These types of actions immediately change the dynamics of the situation and make it more positive.

As with a conversation, if there is something you don't understand, it is better to ask for clarification than to assume you know what he is thinking.

You decide how to react to situations. You choose to be angry or understanding. One reason for many disagreements is unconscious "should" and "must" beliefs. Most people have an idea of how they want their partner to act. However, when you use "should" and "must," your opinions are inflexible, and there isn't room for exceptions. Changing your language to turn your ideas into preferences rather than demands can lower resentment. No matter how much you try, every relationship is going to have conflict sometimes. Learning better communication skills helps you resolve the dispute.

# CHAPTER 14
# Building Assertiveness

You know what you want but usually keep it to yourself. You don't want to make waves or disappoint others, so you remain silent and allow others to take advantage of you. You feel like a pushover. This chapter shows you how to effectively speak up for yourself while remaining respectful of other people. We explain what happens when you aren't assertive, and we explain how to use a few simple steps to speak your mind and let others know what you think and feel.

## Defining Assertiveness

Assertiveness is expressing your needs, wants, beliefs, opinions, and feelings in a way that is respectful to you and others. When you are assertive, you…

- State your point of view.
- Express your feelings.
- Ask for what you want or need.
- Say no without feeling guilty.
- Set boundaries.
- Stand up for yourself and your rights.

Being assertive is not the same as being aggressive. When aggressive, you make demands; when assertive, you ask for what you want.

When you are not assertive, you…

- Say yes even if it is inconvenient, a burden, or unfair to you.
- Have difficulty expressing positive feelings.

- Feel embarrassed or humiliated when criticized.
- Allow people to take advantage of you.
- Go along with the crowd even when you don't agree.
- Become aggressive or angry when someone takes advantage of you.

Some people are naturally more assertive than others; however, it is a learned skill that takes practice.

## Steps for Assertiveness

There are no strict rules for assertiveness; it looks different depending on the person and circumstances. The following steps can help:

*Step 1:* State your point of view. Briefly describe the situation as you see it, including what you expect.

*Step 2:* Discuss how you feel.

*Step 3:* Ask for what you want. Be specific; ask for something measurable, actionable, reasonable, and timely.

*Step 4:* Point out how complying with your preference will benefit everyone involved. Ask for understanding from the other person.

Suppose a close friend invites you to spend the holidays with her and her family. At the last minute, your friend rescinds the invitation because there isn't any room. You feel hurt and angry. You go back and forth. One minute, you want to forcefully tell your friend how you feel; the next, you want to ignore the situation. A better way to handle it is to follow the four steps. Start by calling your friend and setting up a time to talk. Prepare a script outlining what you'd like to say.

*Step 1:* Jill, when you invited me to the holidays, I was excited to be a part of your celebration. I spent time baking cookies and bought small gifts for your family. I didn't make other plans because I was spending the day with you.

*Step 2:* When you canceled our plans, I was hurt and felt that I'm not important to you.

*Step 3:* Next time you invite me to something and you cannot accommodate the invitation, I would prefer that you let me know at least 3 days before, so I have a chance to make other plans.

*Step 4:* I care about you and our relationship. We both must respect each other's time and feelings. Can you understand how I feel?

Being assertive isn't easy, especially if you are used to being passive and staying quiet when others take advantage of you. In the beginning, it is scary. Following a script might help.

A lack of assertiveness could result from one of these problematic thought processes:

- Mind reading. You assume others know what you are thinking and feeling.
- "Should" statements. You assume others should know what you want or expect without you having to express yourself.
- Fortune-telling. You assume the other person won't care about your feelings.
- Catastrophizing. You predict that if you are assertive, it is going to end badly.

## Rights and Responsibilities

It's essential to stand up for your rights, but rights come with responsibilities. Assertiveness requires balancing your needs and rights with those of the people around you. The following table outlines some fundamental rights and the responsibilities that go along with them:

| Rights | Responsibilities |
| --- | --- |
| To be respected | To show respect to others |
| To make choices | To accept the consequences of your choices |
| To make mistakes | To own up to and accept the consequences of your mistakes |
| To express your opinion | To respect that others also have the right to express their opinions, even if you disagree |
| To say no without feeling guilty | To accept no from other people |
| To be honest about your feelings | To not expect others to know how you feel unless you clearly state your feelings |

Your rights could vary depending on the situation. For example, you might not have the right to say no to your boss when given a request, unless it is demeaning or discriminatory or you are willing to lose your job. You do have the right to say no if a friend asks for an inconvenient favor or something that would create a hardship. You choose when to be assertive.

Some people find it hard to say no because they feel guilty or don't want to disappoint someone. However, always saying yes can overload you. Decide on your limits and stick to them. Politely and calmly explain you don't have time right now or the request doesn't fit with your values. Don't apologize and make excuses. Use assertiveness techniques such as rephrasing when the other person isn't willing to accept no the first time.

## When You Aren't Assertive

You are your best advocate. There isn't anyone else who knows what you feel, think, want, and need. If you don't let others know how their actions affect you, chances are they don't know. When you aren't assertive, you frequently end up feeling angry at and resentful toward the other person.

If you aren't assertive, you might…

- Feel embarrassed or humiliated when criticized.
- Develop a need for perfection, so no one has a reason to criticize you.
- Feel you never get what you deserve.
- Resent others for taking advantage of you.
- Have low self-esteem because you think you should stand up for yourself more often.

Being passive or timid affects your life in significant and insignificant ways. At a restaurant, if your food is undercooked or burnt, you eat it anyway because you don't want to bother the server. If you bought something and decided it no longer fit your needs, you give it away or throw it out because you don't want to go back to the store to explain why you no longer want it. Or maybe you've accepted working for years without a raise because you can't bring yourself to request a raise or promotion. No matter what it is, you replay the situation in your mind, thinking about what you could have or should have said and feeling like a failure because you didn't.

Being passive is accepting the other person's terms. When the outcome doesn't matter to you, this is okay. For example, your partner chooses an Italian restaurant, but you wanted Chinese. You don't speak up and think, "We can order Chinese next time." If you didn't mind, there is nothing wrong with accepting someone else's terms. In this case, speaking up and stating you want Chinese food the next time you go out to dinner might work for you. Passive aggression is when you agree, but inside you are resentful. Passive-aggressive behaviors include sarcasm, slamming doors, making cunning remarks, rolling your eyes, or planning retaliation.

## Choosing the Middle Ground

Assertiveness is the middle ground. On one end is passivity; on the other is aggression. Imagine you are standing in line at the grocery store. Someone comes along and jumps in front of you in line. If you react passively, you do nothing. If you respond aggressively, you make a scene. A positive response would be to say, "Excuse me, I was already in line. Could you please move to the end of the line?"

Being overly or regularly passive often leads to resentment and low self-esteem. You go through life wanting to do something but lacking the courage to try. Something always stops you from getting what you want, or maybe you wait for someone or something to push you forward and never taking the first step on your own. When you are passive, other people probably don't know what you want, need, or think.

Aggressiveness is overreacting. An aggressive person uses demands and force—violence or the implied or overt threat of violence—to get what they want. Being aggressive breeds resentment in other people. Assertiveness accepts that your wants, feelings, and needs are valid and that you can stand up for your rights while still treating the other person with respect.

## Helping Others to Be Assertive

Sometimes, other people in your life lack assertiveness, which can lead to frustration and confusion on your part because you want to be responsive to their needs. What they say and do might be contradictory to the previous behavior, or they might not state their needs clearly. One way of overcoming this problem is to help them become more articulate with their needs and desires.

Imagine you and your partner decide to go to the movies. You ask if there is one he wants to see, and the answer is "I don't care, you pick." But when leaving the theatre, he notices a poster for a different movie and says, "I wanted to see that. I wish we had gone to see that one." On the ride home, he is annoyed. You feel frustrated because this has happened before. You might say, "When I ask you what movie you want to see, you say that you don't care but then are annoyed that we do not see the one you wanted. It is frustrating for me. Let's take turns choosing a movie."

# Types of Assertiveness

Assertiveness is standing up for your rights; therefore, being assertive usually requires using "I" statements to let someone know what you think and feel. There are several different ways to use assertiveness.

## Compliments, Praise, and Information

An assertion is not just about complaining or setting boundaries. Compliments and information can be forms of assertiveness. Keep your statements brief and to the point. Don't embellish.

"I enjoyed your presentation."

"I like your new outfit."

"You look nice today."

"I thought you did a great job."

## Self-Disclosure

Stating how you feel sometimes helps to lower the intensity of the emotion or diffuse the situation. Use "I" statements to explain how you feel without attacking the other person.

> "I feel angry."

> "I am nervous about today's presentation."

> "I am unhappy with your behavior."

Body language is an integral part of assertiveness. Your body should be relaxed, and your voice should be neutral. You should stand or sit up straight to reflect confidence. Your arms should be at your sides with your palms open. You should make eye contact. Practice being assertive in front of a mirror. Pay attention to your body language. You want your body to give the same message as your words.

## Empathy

When you have compassion, you show you are aware of someone else's feelings but still expect particular behavior. Showing empathy for the other person's point of view helps lower tendencies toward aggression and gives you time to imagine the other person's position. Pay attention to your tone of voice when using this type of response; it can sound passive-aggressive when delivered with sarcasm.

> "I understand you don't agree with the procedures, but I appreciate that you are willing to complete the job."

> "I understand you are busy but are willing to complete the job by the end of the day."

> "I understand it is your job to tell the boss about my mistakes, but I would prefer it if you tell me first."

## Discrepancy Assertiveness

When there is a discrepancy between what was said previously and what is now occurring or a difference between words and actions, you can resolve it without making accusations; instead, try to clarify information or a misunderstanding.

> "Yesterday, you said you wanted to go out to dinner tonight, but I see you are making dinner. Did something change?"

"You say you don't want a committed relationship but wanting to go out every weekend makes it seem like you want more than a casual relationship. Can you help me understand?"

## Conflict Resolution

Sometimes, stating what you want does not get you what you want. The other person involved has his or her own opinion or side of things. Instead of arguing or feeling as though you cannot get what you want, try negotiating.

Let's say you are on vacation, and your partner wants to spend the day sightseeing, but you want to relax on the beach. You might say, "I understand why it is important for you to see these things, but I'm exhausted today. Can we spend the morning relaxing on the beach and then go to the museum this afternoon?"

Try to figure out a way for both people's needs to be at least partially met.

## Rephrasing Your Assertion

Sometimes, others don't accept your first response and continue to ask the same question or act in the same way toward you. Repeating yourself, possibly several times, is likely to make you frustrated. Instead, ask how you can clarify better or help them to understand your perspective. Suppose a coworker suggests having lunch together.

Coworker: "Do you want to go out to lunch today?"

Response: "No, thank you; I have some errands to do during my lunch hour."

Coworker: "Can't they wait until tomorrow?"

Response: "No, they are important. Can we have lunch tomorrow?"

You can combine this technique with other types of assertiveness, or you can start mildly and become more assertive (but not angry or aggressive) each time the other person doesn't accept your position.

## Consequences

Use this technique as a last resort. Make sure to keep an even tone of voice, relax your body and face, and maintain eye contact, so you do not seem threatening.

"If you continue to ignore my requests, I will need to speak with your supervisor."

Assertiveness is a learned skill and takes practice. Try using the techniques at times you are not emotional, so you get used to speaking up for yourself. Keep a log of when you use one of these strategies. Write down facts about the situation, what you said, and how the other person reacted.

# Acting Assertively

Sometimes, expressing what you want is not enough. You need to act. Following are some examples of how you can act assertively.

You and a friend are out to dinner. You have an early meeting at work and want to go home. Your friend wants to go out for a few more drinks. He insists you come along, despite your objections. You might say, "I know you don't have to work tomorrow, but I do. Thank you for the invitation, but I do need to go home. Good night." Then leave.

You and your roommate walk to class together each morning. She is usually late, and you don't want to arrive after class started. "I can't be late for class again. I will save you a seat." Then go to class.

You are traveling with a friend and are on a tight budget. She wants to go for an expensive dinner and continually insists you should come. You might say, "I am sorry I can't join you. It would be great, but it isn't in my budget. I will meet you back at the hotel. Enjoy your dinner."

You and your partner are arguing. You keep going in circles. You are exhausted and think the discussion is going to go downhill from here. You might say, "I need to pause right now. Can we talk again later when we are both calmer?"

In these examples, you use assertiveness for self-care. When doing so, make sure you are not hurting the other person. Keep your body language calm. It helps to acknowledge the other person's position.

Some tips for practicing assertiveness:

- Politely ask to talk.
- Be aware of your environment; if necessary, ask to talk in private.
- State what you think, feel, and want. Give facts without judging or blaming.
- Speak respectfully. Avoid intimidating or upsetting the other person. Never use violence or the threat of violence.
- Use "I" statements. Never attack the other person.
- Stick to your point, your perspective, and your feelings.
- Remember that no one can make you feel anything. Take responsibility for your feelings.

- Give the other person a chance to voice his or her opinion. Make it a discussion rather than one or both of you trying to win an argument.
- Accept that sometimes the issue can't be resolved, and you must agree to disagree.

Assertiveness, however, is not a guarantee that you get what you want. For example, suppose you ask for a raise at work. You explain why you believe you deserve the raise and point out your achievements. You are assertive. Your boss still might turn you down. Asking does not guarantee the other person reacts according to your wants.

# Accepting Criticism

Criticism is pointing out a mistake, fault, or an area to be improved. It is impossible to go through life without ever receiving negative feedback. You might see criticism as unfavorable or as a judgment against your abilities or against you as a person. Sometimes, though, criticism isn't meant as a negative; it provides the information you can use to grow and learn.

The first step to accepting criticism is to view it as an opportunity to discover how others see you. Suppose your boss sets up a meeting to discuss your work performance. She talks about your strengths but also points out several ways you can improve your performance. She says she noticed you missed details on your last project and would like you to double-check your work. You have two choices: become angry and defensive or consider what your boss said and use the information to become better at your job.

If you have a difficult time accepting criticism, try the following:

- Look for any part of the criticism where you agree. Sometimes you might agree with a fraction of what the other person has said.
- Show empathy by agreeing to that one point.
- Ask for more information on how the other person views that one part.
- Express your point of view with "I" statements.

In the previous example, you might say, "You think sometimes I am careless when completing my work. I agree. Can you give me some guidance to help me improve my work?" By agreeing on one point, you open the possibility of learning and growing in your job.

If you find it hard to respond to criticism on the spot, accept the criticism gracefully. Later, when you have time to think about it, decide what points you want to agree with and take steps to improve those areas. The rest you can simply reject or accept as another person's opinion.

# Misconceptions About Assertiveness

You might be afraid to be assertive and worry about what other people will think of you. It's common to feel that speaking up will elicit adverse reactions. Following are some common misconceptions about assertiveness:

*Misconception:* Being assertive will ruin my relationship.

*Reality:* Assertiveness and setting limits deepens relationships. The other person is usually happier when you set healthy limits and boundaries.

*Misconception:* I will look selfish.

*Reality:* When you are assertive, you stand up for yourself. You put your needs on an equal level with the other person's wants and needs. That doesn't mean you aren't considering another's needs or seeing them as not as necessary as your own. You are merely stating what you feel or want.

*Misconception:* People won't like me.

*Reality:* Think of people you know who are assertive. You might have observed them and wished you were more like them. Are these people unlikeable? Are they respected and well liked? People usually like and respect those who stand up for themselves.

*Misconception:* The other person will get angry.

*Reality:* This is fortune-telling and jumping to assumptions. You are assuming you know how the other person will react and are expecting their reaction will be unreasonable. When you are assertive, you are reasonable, not aggressive.

*Misconception:* I get too nervous about being assertive.

*Reality:* Being assertive, especially if you aren't used to doing so, could make you nervous. Although challenging at first, it becomes more comfortable with time. Start by practicing with people you know well, such as friends and relatives, until you feel comfortable stating your opinion or feelings.

Assertiveness is a give and take. You need to state your opinion and feelings. You also need to take time to actively listen to the other person's point of view. You might get what you want through intimidation, but you gain respect with assertiveness.

Assertiveness is standing up for your rights, wants, and needs by balancing them with the requirements of others. When you are passive, you work with a "you win; I lose" philosophy. When you are aggressive, you operate with the idea, "I win; you lose." When you are assertive, the goal is "I win; you win."

# CHAPTER 15
# Managing Everyday Stress

We live in a fast-paced, high-achievement world. We accept that our days are sometimes stressful. We deal with family and work, find a way to balance both, and still find me time. With everything going on around you, it's hard not to be stressed. In this chapter, you learn what stress is, where it comes from, and how to cope with it.

## What Is Stress?

Stress is an internal pressure you put on yourself. It occurs when faced with overwhelming or challenging situations and signals and you don't think you have the ability or resources to deal with the situation. You feel burdened emotionally or physically. Stress is unique in each person. You might handle certain situations calmly, feeling completely in control, while someone else might feel frazzled.

Stress is unavoidable. From the time you were a child, you learned to deal with it. Short-term pressure can push you to try harder and achieve more. For example, the nervousness you feel before an important test is stress. You study and prepare, but once the exam is over, you feel better. Other times, stress lasts much longer and becomes harmful. Chronic, or long-term, stress can cause frustration and irritability. You might have trouble sleeping, get headaches or stomachaches, have nightmares, or have difficulty concentrating. You feel overwhelmed and unable to handle the situation. Long-term stress is sometimes referred to as *distress* and can be debilitating or deadly. The goal of stress management is to develop coping mechanisms for short-term anxiety and reduce or eliminate long-term stress.

# Identify Your Stressors

Most people juggle several areas of their lives each day, each with its own set of challenges. Some common causes of stress include

- Working long hours
- Pressure to succeed
- Job uncertainty
- Friction with coworkers or supervisors
- Poor working conditions
- Lack of career prospects
- Relationship problems
- Family dysfunction
- Illness
- Financial difficulties
- Moving
- Having a baby
- Starting a job
- Traveling
- Planning a large event

Sometimes, identifying your stressors is easy; you might look at the previous list and quickly see several areas that are stressful for you. Maybe you are working long hours or facing the possibility of losing your job. Perhaps you are going through problems in your relationship and considering divorce. At other times, stressors are harder to figure out. There isn't anything significant going on in your life, but you feel overwhelmed by working, managing your household, or caring for your children. Or maybe your stressors are hiding behind denials, excuses, and assigning blame to others for your problems.

Take time over the next week or two to write down what situations and events cause stress or tension in your life. Note whether this is a one-time event, such as a job interview, or if it is ongoing. For each stressor that is an ongoing situation, place it into a category, such as work, family, illness, pain, or social situations. This helps you identify areas in your life that are causing the most difficulty.

# Problems vs. Problematic Thinking

Once you have a list of everyday stressors, decide whether each is the result of a problem or problematic thinking. Is there a specific problem and a possible solution? If so, sit down and write a plan of action for solving the problem. If it is a result of problematic thoughts, reread Chapter 2. Do you create stress by thinking negatively?

Suppose you wrote down that you feel pressure at work. Your employer laid off some coworkers, and you are worried about your job. You feel the necessity to bring work home because you think any errors or missed deadlines increases your chance of being laid off. Money is tight now, and if the company lays you off, it will get worse. You think…

"I can never get ahead. Something bad always happens."

"I won't be able to pay my bills. It would be terrible if I lose my apartment."

"I should not make any mistakes at work."

"I can't handle this stress."

Some problematic thinking in this example include:

- Catastrophizing ("It would be terrible if I lose my apartment.")
- Overgeneralizing ("I can never get ahead; I can't handle this stress.")
- "Should" and "must" ("I should not make any mistakes at work.")

If you slow down, take some deep breaths, and restructure your thinking, you approach the situation differently. Losing your job presents challenges, but what can you do? Make a list.

Speak with my boss about the possibility of getting laid off. Discuss his expectations of you during this time. Should you take on extra work to make up for people who were already laid off? Ask if there are ways you can improve your performance. Focus on what you can do to minimize potential difficulties. Then reword your concerns:

"If I lose my job, money will be tight. I do have some savings and will be eligible for unemployment to hold me over until I find another job."

"The job I have now is a step up from my previous position, so if I do get laid off, it will be a setback, but I am slowly moving ahead."

"I can work hard and focus on accuracy. Doing my best is what counts."

# Your Turn: Problem Solving

*The form accompanying this exercise is in Appendix C.*

In one or two phrases or sentences, write down a pressing problem you are having. Focus on the actual problem, not how you feel. Writing it down helps you separate fact and emotion.

After you've written your problem, list the possible solutions. Don't worry about whether the answers are practical or realistic right now. Write down all ideas that come to mind. Here's an example.

Problem: Car making a strange noise; needs to be taken to a mechanic.

Solutions:

- Buy a new car.
- Ask a coworker for a ride to work while the vehicle is in the shop.
- Take the bus to work.
- Rent a car until repairs are completed.
- Work from home.
- Take a day off work to take the car to the shop.

Once you have listed all the possible solutions, go back and cross out any unreasonable solutions. You might cross off "buy a new car" because it isn't in your budget and "take the bus to work" because the bus route is inconvenient.

Keep the top two or three solutions, and write down the pros and cons of each one:

*Ask a coworker for a ride to work.*

Pro: least expensive

Con: need to have coworker pick me up, and I don't know if someone is willing to do that.

*Rent a car.*

Pro: gives the most flexibility

Con: might be expensive

*Take a day off work, and take the car to shop.*

Pro: can take the car to shop and wait for repairs

Con: using a vacation day

Now you can decide which choice is best for your situation and create a plan of action. Some problems are more complex. For those, you might need to break your plan of action into steps and work on one step at a time. Monitor your progress and revise as needed until you reach your goal.

# Stress Reduction Strategies

You manage your stress, or it controls you. Stress can contribute to poor physical health, such as heart disease, diabetes, high blood pressure, and stroke. Managing stress improves overall feelings of well-being and increases your longevity. The following are some techniques for managing everyday stress:

*Prioritize.* If you have a long "to-do" list and worry about how to get it all done, take time each morning to prioritize your tasks. Write down everything you want to accomplish. Rate each one. You probably have several tasks on your list that are only mildly important or nonessential. Cross these out. You might have four or five items left. This is your new "to-do" list. Accept that the other tasks might not get done.

*Think in action steps.* Instead of thinking in terms of an entire project from start to finish, break your projects into actionable steps.

*Build an oasis.* When feeling stressed, take a few minutes to build your private retreat. Find a quiet area and take a few deep breaths, or use visualization or positive imagery, as explained in Chapter 6, to imagine yourself in a serene and calm place. As you practice this, you will find it easy to simply close your eyes and go to the quiet space in your mind for a few minutes of peace.

*Determine the probability.* If you tend to catastrophize, take a few minutes to determine the likelihood of your anticipated outcome. Usually, the possibility is much lower than you imagine. Make a list of the steps that would have to occur for your situation to be as catastrophic as you imagined. Assign each step a percentage of how likely it is and multiply all the percentages by each other. The answer is the probability of your outcome occurring.

For example, imagine your boss sent you an email pointing out a problem with one aspect of your performance. You immediately assume you are going to get fired. Look at each event that would lead to that outcome, and realistically evaluate how likely it is to occur.

> I will be on probation. (30 percent chance of occurring)
>
> I will make another mistake. (20 percent chance of occurring)
>
> Multiply those numbers together: (20% + 30%)/2 incidents = 25%

There is a 25 percent chance that you'll get fired, which means there is a 75 percent chance you won't. Most likely, you won't get fired.

List what you can control. Sometimes you feel stress about situations and events you cannot control. Think about what you can manage, and ask yourself if there are concrete steps to take to improve the situation. If there isn't, focus on how to cope with the situation. Remember, even when the situation is out of your control, you can choose your reaction.

*Use relaxation techniques.* In Chapter 7, you learned different relaxation techniques, such as deep breathing and meditation. Focus on relaxing your body.

*Pay attention to negative thought patterns.* Use the list in Chapter 2 to help you identify negative thought patterns and use the ABCD worksheets to come up with more helpful ways of looking at situations.

*Create a stress-coping phrase.* Find a coping phrase you can repeat any time you feel stress. You might use "I feel calm," "I can handle this," or "I am doing the best I can" to silence negative self-talk.

*Make time for yourself.* Schedule time every day for pleasurable activities and relaxation time to help create a balance in your life and put difficult situations into perspective.

*Do a muscle relaxation exercise.* Tighten and relax each muscle in your body for at least 10 seconds. We explain progressive muscle relaxation exercises in Chapter 7. Learn your body's stress signals. Paying attention to how your body reacts to stress, such as tight muscles, helps you identify stress early and take steps to change your perspective.

*Ask for help.* When your stress continues to build despite your attempts to reduce it, you might need help. If you have a hard time with this, review the assertion strategies in Chapter 14.

*Schedule a tech-free break.* Shut the cell phone off and just tune out. In today's busy world with cell phones, tablets, email, and social media, it can be hard to take a break. Your mind is continually churning, and you are always checking for the next email, text, or post. Schedule an hour, a day, or a weekend to shut off your electronic devices and rejuvenate.

## Your Turn: Create a Stress Worksheet

*The form accompanying this exercise is in Appendix C.*

Create a worksheet to complete when you feel overwhelmed. Your sheet should have the following:

- What is the situation?
- What is my immediate reaction?
- What emotion am I feeling?
- Evidence to support distressing thoughts.
- Evidence to disprove distressing thoughts.
- Balanced statement.
- What emotion am I now feeling?

Answer each with a few words or sentences. When filling in your worksheet, remember, you can describe emotions and moods in one or two words. Thoughts are more complex and might require phrases or sentences.

# Exercise Your Stress Away

Regular exercise reduces stress levels. It releases muscle tension and gives you a chance to break the cycle of negative and stressful thoughts. Some people find activity to be a form of mindfulness meditation. They get "in the zone" and forget about problems for a short time. During exercise, your body produces endorphins, sometimes called the "feel-good" brain chemical. Some research shows exercise might change how your brain releases and uses chemicals, making the effects of exercise on stress last long after you have stopped.

When beginning an exercise program...

- Talk to your doctor, especially if you have any health conditions. Be sure exercise is safe and ask what types of activities are best.
- Schedule exercise into your daily routine. Other tasks and responsibilities might seem more important, but remember, exercise helps you better manage stress and can improve cognitive performance and memory.
- Find the right exercise program for you. Choose something you like to do. You are more likely to stick with an exercise program if it fits into your lifestyle. Consider your time and budget.

According to the U.S. Centers for Disease Control and Prevention, adults should have a minimum of two and a half hours of moderate aerobic exercise per week (150 minutes). Spread this out throughout the week based on what is best for you. You can break daily routines into several sessions each day, as long as each exercise session is at least 10 minutes long. If you don't already exercise, start small. Even 10 minutes of exercise each day has been found to lower stress levels.

Everyone feels stress at some point in their lives. It occurs when you don't believe you can handle a situation. Proactively looking at your triggers and coming up with coping actions and statements provides you with a way to better manage stressful situations. Other activities, such as deep breathing, progressive muscle relaxation, meditation, and exercise, can also reduce levels of stress.

# PART 4

# CBT for Specific Conditions and Situations

Research shows that CBT is an effective way to manage mental and physical health conditions. People using CBT techniques often reduce or eliminate the need for medication in their treatment. CBT provides lasting change and gives you the skills you need to continue your progress, even after your CBT sessions are completed.

In this part, we address how CBT helps you manage depression, anxiety, obsessive-compulsive disorder, and some physical illnesses. Choose areas you find most problematic in your life first; however, you might find useful information in the other chapters as well. Please note some of the issues discussed in this section are medical issues, and you should consult with your doctor or therapist if you need additional help. You can use the CBT techniques in this book in conjunction with outside therapy.

# CHAPTER 16
# Overcoming Depression

Depression affects about 1 in 10 adults in the United States. You might think of it as feeling blue or sad, but it is much more than that. People living with depression frequently feel helpless and hopeless about their futures. In this chapter, you'll learn how to recognize signs of depression and the negative thought processes that contribute to depression. You'll learn how to stop the cycle of negative thoughts and how caring for your physical needs can lessen feelings of depression.

## Sadness vs. Depression

Everyone feels sad at some time in their lives; it is a normal human reaction when faced with loss or disappointment. Sadness, although painful, is temporary. Depression, however, can last for weeks, months, or years. There is more to depression than sadness.

Consider these critical differences between sadness and depression:

- Sadness is usually a result of circumstances.
- Depression does not always have a rational or logical cause.
- Sadness temporarily reduces your ability to enjoy parts of your life, but you are usually still able to cope and participate in activities.
- Depression typically lasts longer, is more intense, and is often debilitating. It interferes with your ability to function and care for yourself.
- Sadness is not constant. You can have interspersed moments of laughter.
- Depression can be chronic; it is something you experience almost daily for at least half of the day.
- Sadness fades with time or once your problem is resolved.
- Depression usually does not resolve itself without some type of intervention.

According to the U.S. Centers for Disease Control and Prevention, approximately 1 in 10 people seek medical help for symptoms of depression. Women are more likely to have depression than men, as are people who live below the poverty line and those between the ages of 40 and 59.

While profound sadness is one of the symptoms of depression, there are other symptoms:

- Lack of interest in activities you previously enjoyed
- Changes in appetite—either overeating or loss of appetite
- Agitation and irritability
- Insomnia or sleeping too much
- Loss of energy or fatigue
- Trouble concentrating
- Indecisiveness
- Feelings of hopelessness or worthlessness
- Thoughts of death or suicide

Sadness is a normal human emotion; depression is an illness—you can't "snap out of it." If you are depressed and have trouble caring for yourself, not connecting with others in your relationships, or experiencing some of the symptoms listed, you should speak with your doctor.

# The Role of CBT in Treating Depression

Research shows CBT is effective in treating mild and moderate depression. CBT techniques work to…

- Change negative thought patterns and replace them with positive, balanced ways of looking at situations and events.
- Stop ruminations.
- Schedule activities.
- Overcome shame and hopelessness.

While CBT is sometimes used alone as a treatment for depression, your doctor might recommend medication combined with CBT. Talk with your doctor, discuss treatment options, and together decide which is best for you.

In CBT, the term *cognitive triad* refers to depressive thoughts in three areas:

1. Thoughts about yourself: I am a failure; I am unlovable; I have no control.

2. Thoughts about the world or situations you face: The world is cruel; this situation is unfair.

3. Thoughts about the future: My future is hopeless and bleak.

Dr. Aaron Beck, the founder of CBT, first proposed the concept of the cognitive triad based on the idea that depressive disorders use negative views of yourself, your life experience, the world around you, and your future as the foundation for your perspective.

Suppose you recently went through a painful breakup. If you are prone to depression, your thoughts might be similar to the following:

1. I am not loveable. I can't cope with this. I am alone.

2. This is entirely unfair. He/she hurt me without reason.

3. I will never be happy again. I will never find love.

These types of thoughts…

1. Ignore the fact that you have friends and family to support you during this time, and you have coped with difficult situations in the past.

2. Blame your ex rather than considering that both of you wanted different things out of the relationship, and you are now free to find someone whose relationship goals more closely match yours. You fail to take any responsibility for the problems in the relationship.

3. Assume there is no one else out there for you. Assume no one will want to stay with you long-term. Believe you won't find happiness again. Assume you need another person to survive.

You can use the ABC chart to think more realistically. While you will probably still feel sad over the end of the relationship, you understand it is temporary.

| A: Activating Event | B: Thoughts or Beliefs | C: Coping Thoughts |
| --- | --- | --- |
| Breakup | I am not loveable. | I frequently meet people who enjoy spending time with me. |
| | I can't cope with this. I am alone. | I have friends who can help me through this time. |
| | This is entirely unfair. | Not every relationship will be forever. |

*continues…*

| A: Activating Event | B: Thoughts or Beliefs | C: Coping Thoughts |
|---|---|---|
| | He/she hurt me without reason. | We were not a good fit because we wanted different things from the relationship. |
| | I will never be happy again. | I feel sad, but I have felt sad before, and it was temporary. |
| | I will never find love. | "Never" is a strong word. It is improbable that I will *never* find love. |
| | I can't cope. | I have coped with difficult situations before and can deal with this. |

# The "Do Nothing" Syndrome

One of the hallmark symptoms of depression is lack of motivation. You might withdraw from family and friends and struggle to get out of bed each day. You might stop going to work or spending time on hobbies. You could put off household chores or responsibilities. These behaviors often make you feel worse. When you stop "doing," you feel useless and hopeless.

One of the goals of CBT is to gradually increase your level of activity. For example, if you have been spending your days in bed, it is unreasonable to assume that one day you are only going to get up and be active all day. But you can set realistic goals for activity and build on them. On the first day, you might set a goal of getting out of bed and taking a shower. It is essential to start your goals from where you are now, not from where you think you should be.

Create a daily activity schedule. Planning activities increases your motivation to follow through. The following example breaks the day into 1 or 2 hour increments. Make a list of pursuits you feel you can do now and those that you previously enjoyed. Rate them from most comfortable to hardest; for example, you might put "take a walk" and rate this as easy, and you might put "meet a friend for lunch" and rate this as difficult. When you start creating a schedule, start with easy tasks.

| Time | Activity |
|---|---|
| 8–9 A.M. | Get up and shower |
| 9–10 A.M. | Have breakfast |
| 10–11 A.M. | Rest |
| 11–noon | Straighten the house |
| Noon–1 P.M. | Eat lunch |

| | |
|---|---|
| 1–2 P.M. | Rest |
| 2–3 P.M. | Read |
| 3–4 P.M. | Rest |
| 4–5 P.M. | Pleasure activity: Go to the dog park |
| 5–6 P.M. | Have dinner |
| 6–7 P.M. | Watch television |
| 7–8 P.M. | Watch television |
| 8–9 P.M. | Read |
| 9–10 P.M. | Go to bed |

Each day or every few days, substitute a pleasurable activity with rest or reading time. Don't overload your schedule; you could get overwhelmed and give up. The goal of creating a plan is to become more active gradually. Keep a notebook with your daily plan so you can monitor your progress.

# Avoidance

It might be tempting to fill your schedule with activities that take the place of going out of the house. Suppose you fill your daily agenda with "read" or "watch television." If you haven't gotten out of bed, adding these activities is a good start, if you get out of bed to do them. However, they could be your way of avoiding other more challenging activities, such as those that require leaving the house. Avoidance might cause you to feel worse than before because you feel isolated and alone.

What activities did you leave off your schedule? Review the following list and check the items you are avoiding:

❏ Seeing friends

❏ Answering the phone or responding to texts

❏ Looking at or answering emails

❏ Household chores and responsibilities (cleaning, paying bills, and so on)

❏ Hygiene (showering, bathing, washing clothes)

❏ Taking part in hobbies

❏ Going to work

Look over your list. Do you have avoidance behaviors? Try to switch one avoidance behavior for a healthy behavior each day. Review the following example and then choose one avoidance behavior you use and fill in the information.

*Avoidance Behavior:* Not seeing friends.

*Effects:* I feel isolated and more depressed.

*Alternate Behavior:* I can get together with a friend once a week.

*Benefits:* I get out of the house. I have the support of my friends. I don't feel isolated.

*Obstacles:* Most of my friends work full time, and many have families as well. It is hard for them to find the time.

*Steps:* Maybe it is better if I meet a friend for lunch and choose a place close to her job, so it does not take much time from her other responsibilities. I will text friends to see who is available.

*Your turn:*

*Avoidance Behavior:*

*Effects:*

*Alternate Behavior:*

*Benefits:*

*Obstacles:*

*Steps:*

Some people with depression shy away from friends and family because they think, "I am not good company right now." You might worry you have nothing to say or your despair will be front and center during the lunch. You choose who you text. Think about who is supportive and understanding, and during lunch, explain what you feel comfortable sharing about your situation and ask for their support.

# Ruminations

Rumination is a hallmark behavior for people with depression. Ruminating is when your thoughts play in a continuous loop. You repeat the same scene. You can't shut off the thoughts. Ruminations often center around the following:

- What if…?
- If only….
- How did this happen?
- Why me?
- Why do I feel this way?

- Why didn't I do things differently?
- I feel bad; I am always going to feel this way; I am hopeless.

Ruminations are all-consuming. Once you begin, you can't stop. You might find that you have been sitting and thinking about something for hours on end without realizing how much time passed.

When you notice the loop starting, write down the time, where you are, and what you are thinking. Keep track for a few days and use this information to help you break the habit of ruminating. For example, you might find that you ruminate in the morning when you are still lying in bed. You start thinking about a troubling situation and realize that you have been lying in bed for an hour, going over the same thoughts. Or you might lie awake at night, ruminating about the problems of the day.

It takes a conscious decision to break the chain of thoughts to stop ruminating. Don't worry about the content; it is the process of rumination you want to stop. Make a list of activities you can do whenever you find yourself ruminating. Your list might include the following:

- Exercise for 15 minutes
- Do a mindfulness meditation exercise
- Read a magazine or book
- Do a puzzle
- Do a breathing exercise

Choose one item from the list and make that your "go-to" activity to stop the circle of thoughts. Be sure the activities on your list occupy your mind and don't allow your mind to wander. The idea is to provide you with alternative thoughts. The more absorbed you are, the more likely your ruminations stop. Become mindful in your activity of choice; concentrate fully on the task instead.

# Your Turn: Reduce Your Ruminations

*The form accompanying this exercise is in Appendix C.*

To help reduce rumination, make a list of current issues in your life. List your thoughts in all three areas: yourself, the world, and your future. Then, come up with a coping statement in response to each problem.

Your list might look like this:

*Career*

>**Myself:** I hate my job.
>
>**The world or situation:** Everyone is out for themselves in my company.
>
>**Future:** I will never be successful.

*Finance*

>**Myself:** I am stuck in a low-paying job and have no money. I should have gone to college.
>
>**The world or situation:** Everyone makes more money than me.
>
>**Future:** I am never going to have the money to retire.

*Social Life*

>**Myself:** I have no friends. I am too shy.
>
>**The world or situation:** No one wants to hang out with me.
>
>**Future:** I cannot make friends because of my shyness.

These are negative and unhelpful thoughts. Repeating them in your mind makes you feel worse and stops you from finding solutions The following steps can help you challenge your negative thought processes.

*Step One:* Use the ABCD method to label and challenge your negative thoughts.

*Step Two:* Use behavior experiments, as explained in Chapter 10, to challenge and find solutions.

Your new list of thoughts would look like this:

*Career*

>**Myself:** I don't like what I am doing at work, but it gives me a steady income.
>
>**The world or situation:** No one at work seems to have time to train me on the new software. Maybe there is online training, or I could suggest taking on a few extra tasks in exchange for someone's time.
>
>**Future:** I am going to look into taking college classes online or at a local college.

*Finance*

>**Myself:** I have enough money right now to pay my necessary bills. If I get a second job or do freelance work, I could have some extra cash.

**The world or situation:** Everyone's situation is different. What other people do or do not have has nothing to do with me. I can focus on myself.

**Future:** I can start a retirement account and put a small amount away each week.

*Social Life*

**Myself:** I get along well with the people at work.

**The world or situation:** I know people get busy with their own lives.

**Future:** I can start by asking someone to join me at lunch instead of eating alone at my desk. I can bring my lunch but eat in the cafeteria with my coworkers.

*Step Three:* Select one area to work on first. When you feel satisfied with your progress in that area, move to a different one. Some considerations when choosing what to work on include, what is easiest, what would provide the quickest benefit, or what could help me solve multiple problems.

*Step Four:* Create coping statements—short, one-sentence statements that challenge your negative self-talk. Often when you are depressed, you become critical of yourself. A coping statement is a powerful tool to manage depression. Come up with specific thoughts that sum up a positive point of view.

| Negative Thought | Coping Statement |
| --- | --- |
| I am upset about my career. | I am a smart, capable person. It takes time to build the career I want, but I have a plan. |
| I am upset about money. | I can live an abundant life in many ways. |
| I am upset about my social life. | I am a likable, accepting, and friendly person. |

# Take Care of Yourself

When depressed, you might stop caring about yourself and your environment. Some people overeat; some barely eat. Some forego taking a shower; others might wear the same clothes for several days. The mind and body are connected; if you ignore your physical body, you can't expect your mind to feel good. Hygiene, exercise, proper nutrition, and sleep play a vital role in treating depression.

## Diet

There isn't a specific "depression" diet. There isn't a miracle food that is going to make you feel better suddenly. However, creating and sticking to a well-balanced meal plan is essential. You should be eating three meals (or five smaller meals) every day. Your diet should include fruits, vegetables, whole grains, and protein. If you are eating mostly junk food, start replacing sweets with fruits or whole-grain snacks.

When depressed, avoid caffeine, alcohol, excessive sugar, and refined carbohydrates. These foods can make you feel better temporarily but generally reduce your energy in the long term.

## Exercise

Numerous studies show that exercise improves mood and feelings of well-being. For some people, exercise works as well as antidepressants in treating depression. It reduces stress and helps you sleep better at night.

Cardio exercises such as brisk walking, jogging, jumping rope, and bike riding raise your heart rate and improve your mood. If you go to a gym, try the elliptical trainer, stationary bike, or brisk walking or jogging on the treadmill. You might also consider joining a class that raises your heart rate, such as Zumba or aerobics. Other types of exercises, such as stretching, yoga, and Pilates, can help you to relax.

If you're not exercising now, remember to start small and check with your doctor first. Begin with 10 minutes a day and work your way up to 30 minutes of exercise several times per week. The recommended amount of activity is 150 minutes per week for adults. If you have trouble motivating yourself, ask a friend to join you. Exercising with someone could give you the motivation to keep going.

## Sleep

Sleep disturbances are one symptom of depression. Some people have insomnia, while others sleep too much. Most adults need between 7 and 9 hours of sleep each night. Use your daily schedule to plan the time you go to bed and what time you wake up. Avoid sleeping at other times. Not getting enough sleep can cause symptoms of depression to worsen. Without the proper amount of sleep, you can feel irritable, anxious, and depressed. You might find it hard to concentrate or have impaired memory and judgment.

The following are tips to help you sleep better:

- Go to bed and get up at the same time each day. Even if you have nothing to do, get out of bed each morning at the same time—plan sleeping times in your daily schedule.
- Reduce the stimuli around you about 1 hour before bedtime. Lower the lights or turn them off, turn down the volume on the television, turn off your computer, and put down your phone.

- Spend an hour before bedtime engaged in a relaxing activity. Read a book, take a warm bath or shower, knit, or write in a journal. Get into bed only when you are ready to go to sleep.
- Write down everything you are worried about in a "worry journal." Then put the journal aside. Giving yourself a specific time each day to worry allows you to "put aside your worries" and clears your mind.
- Avoid caffeine after 1 P.M. If you find you can't sleep, eliminate caffeine and then slowly add it back.
- Don't exercise right before bed, as this can interfere with sleep. If you prefer working out in the evening, go straight to the gym after work and then relax for the rest of the evening.
- Reserve the bedroom for sleep and intimacy with your partner. Don't spend time in bed eating, reading, or watching TV.
- Create a relaxing environment in your bedroom. Make it a comfortable place.
- Use white noise, such as a fan or sound machine, to help you sleep.

The relaxation techniques discussed in Chapter 6 might also help improve your sleep. As you become more active during the day, learn to combat negative thoughts or stop ruminating, and vrest might naturally come easier.

Sadness is a temporary reaction to an unpleasant situation or loss. Depression is a complex illness with many possible causes, such as deficiencies in mood regulation in the brain, genetic predisposition, traumatic or stressful events, physical illness, or as a side effect of medication. When you have depression, you can't "snap out of it." Changing negative thought processes helps some people reduce or eliminate symptoms of depression.

# CHAPTER 17
# Dealing with Anxiety Disorders

We are all familiar with the "butterflies in the stomach" feeling. It happens when we feel nervous, such as before a test, a speech, starting a new job, or going on a first date. These feelings are intense but usually short lived; once the event is over, the feeling goes away. Everyone feels nervous from time to time, but if anxiety becomes overwhelming and interferes with your ability to function, it could be a sign of an anxiety disorder. There are different types of anxiety disorders, each with some unique symptoms or triggers. In this chapter, you learn about the different kinds of anxiety and CBT strategies to help you cope.

## Types of Anxiety Disorders

The term *anxiety disorder* encompasses different kinds of anxiety; collectively, anxiety disorders are one of the most common types of mental illness, with 18 percent of adults in the United States experiencing symptoms each year.

Each type has unique characteristics; however, there are some common symptoms:

- Trouble sleeping
- Overpowering fear
- Repeated thoughts
- Frequent worrying
- Avoiding specific places or situations

Physical symptoms include a pounding heart, shortness of breath, muscle tension, and stomachaches.

Common types of anxiety disorders include:

*Social Anxiety Disorder:* You are often afraid of participating in social interactions. You worry about looking foolish or stupid. You believe other people judge you, and you worry about being laughed at or humiliated. You are self-conscious. If someone offers you criticism, you are devastated.

*Generalized Anxiety Disorder:* You worry excessively about everyday problems or what could happen in the future. You frequently have a feeling of impending doom and are sure something terrible will happen. Your worry distracts you from your responsibilities and keeps you awake at night. Even though you know it is irrational or exaggerated, you can't stop yourself from worrying.

*Panic Disorder:* You have a sudden feeling of terror. Your heart races; you gasp for air; and you feel nauseous, lightheaded, dizzy, shaky, and sweaty. You think you are going crazy or that it is a heart attack. The intense feelings typically last about 10 to 15 minutes. You avoid places or situations because you are afraid of having another panic attack.

*Post-Traumatic Stress Disorder (PTSD):* You went through a traumatic event. It could have been war, being a victim of or witnessing a crime, sexual assault, abuse, a serious accident, or a natural disaster. You have flashbacks, nightmares, and sometimes feel detached from life. You are often irritable, have mood swings, and are hypervigilant about your surroundings. You avoid places, people, and situations that remind you of the event.

*Phobias:* You have an excessive and irrational fear of a particular object or situation. It could be a fear of flying, dogs, heights, bridges, injections, or water—or it could be something else entirely. Your anxiety disrupts and limits your life because you avoid places where you might encounter the feared object or situation.

## The Role of CBT in Treating Anxiety Disorders

As with depression, there are several treatment options for anxiety disorders. CBT is the most-used type of therapy for treating anxiety. You can use the strategies in this book as a self-help program, or you can use them in conjunction with other treatments, such as medication.

When using CBT to treat anxiety, the goals include…

- Learning to spot early warning signs of anxiety.
- Lowering symptoms and managing physical sensations.
- Reducing avoidance of situations necessary to your life.
- Challenging how you perceive problems.
- Developing a sense of internal control and a tolerance for uncertainty.

- Building resilience when faced with stress and discomfort.
- Accepting challenges with confidence.

Pay attention to how your body and mind react to anxiety to "catch" it in the early stages when CBT techniques can better disarm it. Throughout this chapter, we explain different strategies to use. At first, you might not know where to start. That's okay. Take your time and experiment with different techniques to find what works best for you. Once you find the right combination, you can implement them when you feel the first signs of anxiety.

# Facing Fears

Right now, you might go to great lengths to avoid feeling anxious. For example, you might drive out of your way to avoid crossing a bridge or spend 20 hours driving to avoid flying. You might cross the street to steer clear of a dog or turn down a job because it is on the 20th floor, and you are afraid of riding in elevators. When you allow fears such as these to control your life, you limit yourself and take away opportunities to confront and overcome them.

*Exposure therapy* is when you face your fears in small steps. It works in person, through virtual simulation or by merely viewing images. Frequently, these methods are combined; for example, you might start exposure therapy by looking at pictures, move on to a virtual depiction using videos or computer-based images, and finally confront your fears in person. When gradually exposed, it is called *graded therapy*. Other types of exposure therapy are called *flooding exposure* or *systematic desensitization*.

*Flooding exposure* is typically only used with in-person exposures, and it exposes you to the feared object or situation for a prolonged amount of time until you no longer feel anxiety. *Systematic desensitization* is graded exposure combined with relaxation exercises. You use a technique such as deep breathing before and during each step.

During graded exposure, you repeatedly expose yourself to the feared object or situation. Each step purposely triggers your anxiety. The desire to stop and avoid the uncomfortable feelings is high, but it is essential to stick with it, letting your fear peak and subside. This type of therapy works if you repeat the same step until your anxiety is manageable. Moving too quickly through stages or stopping while you still feel anxious reinforces fears. The goal is to tolerate a situation without feeling the need to run away.

Suppose you are afraid of dogs. You don't visit friends if you know they have dogs, and you have stopped taking walks after dinner because several neighbors walk their dogs then. Any time you see or hear a dog, you start shaking, and fear overwhelms you.

Suppose your end goal is visiting friends who own a dog. Think about the steps needed to reach that goal. In Chapter 5, Setting Goals, you learned how to create a ladder, with each rung representing one step. Your end goal is the top rung of your ladder, the more manageable steps on the bottom.

| Step | Goal |
|---|---|
| 15 | Visit your friend with a dog. |
| 14 | Pet a dog off a leash. |
| 13 | Pet a dog on a leash. |
| 12 | Pet a small dog someone is holding. |
| 11 | Stand next to a dog off a leash. |
| 10 | Stand next to a dog on a leash. |
| 9 | Have a dog off a leash across the room. |
| 8 | Have a dog on a leash across the room. |
| 7 | Sit in a room with a dog outside in the backyard. |
| 6 | See a dog across the street. |
| 5 | Hear a dog bark. |
| 4 | Watch videos of dogs. |
| 3 | Look at pictures of big dogs. |
| 2 | Imagine a dog that scares you. |
| 1 | Imagine a dog you think is cute. |

Begin with step one and repeat it daily until you don't feel anxious. This step could take one, two, or more days. Take your time and focus on the level until you feel comfortable. Only then should you move to the second step.

Use relaxation skills to reduce the physical feelings of anxiety. It is normal to want to take a break when the tension becomes uncomfortable, but resist the urge to stop. The goal is to tolerate the anxiety. Practice deep breathing or muscle relaxation while you are completing the step. The purpose of exposure therapy is for you to accept that you might feel anxious, but remember these feelings are temporary and won't hurt you. Continue with each step using the same process.

Sometimes, the steps might include increasing the time exposed to your trigger. For example, suppose you are working to overcome a fear of heights, and your end goal is to stand on a balcony. An excellent first step is to stand in the doorway and look out. Next, you can take one step outside. Then, you can walk over to the railing. When you reach that point, set goals to increase how long you stay out. Exposure therapy works because each exposure increases your sense of control over the situation, which decreases your anxiety.

Before starting an exposure exercise, practice relaxation skills you learned in Chapter 6, so you can begin each step in a relaxed state.

Track your progress as you work your way up the ladder. Some people find it helpful to rate their fear. For example, "On day one, my fear was at an 8 out of 10." If you prefer, you can use ratings such as "very," "somewhat," "a little," or "not at all." The point is to see your progression. When you look back and see you used the word "very" on the first day, but now you rate your fear as "somewhat," you can see your progress, which motivates you to continue.

## Your Turn: Expose Yourself

Write down several situations or objects that make you anxious. Start with the one you believe is simplest to overcome.

Create an end goal—how you would behave if you did not have this fear.

Break your goal down into steps. There is no rule on how many you should have, but try to create at least 5 to 10. Choose a relaxation technique to use before each exposure.

## Turn Worry into Problem Solving

One of the main symptoms of generalized anxiety disorder is the endless worry. You know your concern is irrational, but you feel powerless to stop. You worry about everything. You imagine every possible outcome—and usually, they are all disastrous.

Worry is never helpful, but problem solving is. Whenever you catch yourself worrying about something, write it down, and reword it as a problem to solve. For example, you are worried because you don't have enough money to cover your bills. You imagine being evicted, living on the street, or being hungry. Now, turn this around.

*Problem:* I need an additional $300.00 each month to cover my bills.

*Possible Solutions:*

- Get a second job. (these are complete sentences)
- Review my bills to see where I can cut expenses.

Now, choose a solution and create steps to solve your problem. (Your example could have several more solutions.)

If you worry about things or situations that can't be solved or you have no control over, try to redirect your attention. Find an activity you can do for 15 minutes to occupy your mind. Be mindful, which brings you to the present moment. Worry is about the future; mindfulness is about the present.

# Accepting Uncertainty

Some people have a high tolerance for uncertainty. They relish the idea of the unexpected and look forward to finding out what life has to offer. Others feel agitated about the unknown. It is normal to be curious about the future, but they want to know every detail: What is going to happen, and when it is going to happen?

If you have a low tolerance for uncertainty, you probably worry incessantly. You might try to control events and people to eliminate the uncertainty. Still, because you can't possibly know beforehand what is going to happen, it is crucial to learn to live with uncertainty. People with a low tolerance for ambiguity, might...

- Procrastinate or avoid situations that can't be controlled or that have a high level of uncertainty.
- Always seek reassurance from others.
- Be indecisive.
- Have a hard time delegating.
- End relationships.
- Avoid challenges.

You try to control things and events around you to create the future you believe should occur. You don't want to leave the future up to chance. But, trying to control the future takes a lot of time and energy and often leaves you exhausted and frustrated.

One way to lessen uncertainty fears is to use a backward CBT approach. Begin with behaviors instead of thoughts. Once you change a single action and realize that the situation turned out okay, you learn that uncertainty is okay. For example, try delegating the planning for an upcoming activity to someone else. When it is over, ask yourself: Did things turn out okay, even though I didn't know what was going to happen? If something didn't turn out, how did I cope with the situation? Was it as bad as I imagined?

Living with uncertainty takes practice. People who have a high tolerance for ambiguity have learned that no matter the outcome—good or bad—they can cope with the situation. As you practice, it gets easier.

# Your Turn: Create a Worry Script

A worry script is a type of exposure therapy using a scenario that hasn't occurred. It sometimes helps to relieve fears of the future. Think about something you are worried about happening in the future. For example, you might worry about your children or significant other having a car accident. What is the worst possible scenario? Fill in details: what the scene looks like, what you hear, and how you feel. Write using all five of your senses.

Every day for 2 weeks, write about the same scene. Don't write the same words; look at it from a different perspective. For example, one day, you write what the scene physically looks like; on another day, you might write about your emotions. You might feel upset or even start to worry more about the situation. This is all normal; just continue to write about it every day.

At the end of 2 weeks, you should feel less anxious when you rewrite the script. You might feel and think that writing about something makes it happen; if it does occur, you somehow caused it. This is known as *magical thinking*. Rationally, you know thinking about something does not cause it to occur. You know life doesn't work that way. This exercise exposes you to a situation you fear to reduce your emotional response to it. It doesn't mean that your feelings for your family have lessened.

# Your Turn: Managing Big Problems

*The form accompanying this exercise is in Appendix C.*

Anxiety occurs when you perceive you are unable to cope with a situation. The following steps help you work through your thoughts and feelings.

*Step 1:* Write down your perception of the problem.

*Step 2:* Write down your perception of your ability to cope.

*Step 3:* Identify your problematic thought processes using the list in Chapter 2.

*Step 4:* Restructure your thoughts to show a more balanced view of the situation.

*Step 5:* Focus on your new balanced attitude.

Let's look at how these steps can be applied. Imagine you are worried about your relationship. You and your partner are going through a rocky period. You worry that you could get a divorce. You ruminate about any disagreement, no matter how small. You don't think you can emotionally cope with a divorce.

*Step 1:* Write down your perception of the problem.

> My partner and I have been disagreeing a lot lately. I think we will get a divorce.

*Step 2:* Write down your perception of your ability to cope.

> I cannot cope with a divorce. I can't be alone.

*Step 3:* Identify your problematic thought processes using the list in Chapter 2.

- Overgeneralizing and catastrophizing: We will get a divorce; I can't be alone.
- Mind reading: I am making assumptions about my partner's feelings about the disagreements.
- Black-and-white thinking: I assume we either have a good marriage or we are getting a divorce. I don't see any in between or recognize that relationship problems are often temporary.

*Step 4:* Restructure your thoughts to show a more balanced view of the situation.

> I have no idea how my partner feels other than what they tell me.
>
> Many relationships have ups and downs. Every disagreement does not point to divorce.
>
> Even if we do get divorced, I can manage. I will be sad, but I am capable of living on my own.

*Step 5:* Focus on your new, balanced attitude.

> Disagreements are a normal part of a relationship. It is impossible to know what my partner thinks and feels about an argument unless I ask and listen. Even so, disagreeing does not mean divorce, and if my marriage did fall apart, I am capable and will manage.

Excessive worrying is the result of trying to solve problems before they occur. Make sure you are working to solve actual issues, not those you imagine. Using mindfulness helps. Allow your thoughts about potential problems travel across your mind without searching for a solution. Merely accept that it is your thought. Remind yourself that living with uncertainty is a part of life, and you can find a solution if and when the problem arises.

# Behavior Assignments

Uncertainty, ambiguity, and discomfort increase anxiety. The next time you feel anxious, try to unravel your thoughts and feelings about the situation. Focus on determining when and where the ideas appear. Create a new attitude or reword it as a behavior assignment for yourself. Use the following examples as templates for creating your behavior assignments.

## Avoiding Discomfort

*Situation:* If I get on the subway, I will have a panic attack. That will be awful and embarrassing. I can't take the subway.

*Catching your negative thoughts:* I am anxious because I am trying to avoid discomfort. This is fortune-telling; I am not sure I will have a panic attack. It is also mind reading because I am assuming other people will judge me.

*New thoughts:* When I get on the subway, my heart starts racing. I might have a panic attack, but I can use deep breathing and mindfulness to calm myself. If I do have one, people around me are usually helpful and kind, not judgmental. I might not have a panic attack.

*Behavior assignment:* I will get on the subway, get off at the next stop, and keep reminding myself that I can cope with this.

## Uncertainty

*Situation:* My daughter has applied to several colleges. I am anxious about what is going to happen and am worried that she isn't going to be accepted, even though she is a good student. She is going to be devastated.

*Catching your negative thoughts:* I am worried about something that hasn't yet happened and most likely won't happen. I can address the problem if she doesn't get accepted, but right now, there isn't a problem to solve. I am fortune-telling. I am also catastrophizing because I assume she won't get accepted at any college.

*New thoughts:* She applied to several colleges. She has excellent grades and is an active student. Now that she sent the applications, we need to sit back and wait.

*Behavior assignment:* I need to consider different options. If she doesn't get accepted into her first choice, there are other good schools around. She could also take a year off to do volunteering work and improve her resumé.

Paying attention to your physical and emotional signs of anxiety helps you "catch" it early and use CBT techniques to lessen your symptoms. Exposure therapy is one such technique and is particularly helpful when you have specific anxieties, such as a fear of dogs. Strategies for anxiety usually work best when you break your goal into small manageable steps.

# CHAPTER 18
# Controlling Anger

Anger is a normal human response to a perceived threat or wrongdoing on someone else's part. It is energizing, and when used constructively, it helps you right a wrong. When used destructively, anger eats away at your self-confidence and creates problems in your life. This chapter helps you to determine if your anger is healthy or unhealthy and provides strategies to lower your anger levels.

## What Is Anger?

The term anger encompasses feelings from annoyance to full-blown rage. It is a normal human emotion that everyone feels from time to time. It can occur when you feel stressed or when someone infringes on your rights, threatens you, disappoints you, or takes advantage of you. Anger gives you a burst of energy and can propel you to make positive changes in your life; but it can also create problems in relationships and at work.

## Understanding Your Anger

Every day, things happen, and you might feel your anger flare—your boss asks you to stay late to finish a report when you have plans, your partner doesn't take the trash out, a driver cuts you off, or a cashier is rude. It's easy to assume these events caused you to become angry. However, it is not the events themselves that made you mad; it is your interpretation of the situation that caused the anger. Each of us has core beliefs, which drive our automatic thoughts, as discussed in Chapter 3. These thoughts influence your reaction to the event. By identifying and changing those thoughts and core beliefs, you can choose your response to lessen feelings of anger.

## Your Turn: Creating an Anger Log

*The form to accompanying this exercise is in Appendix C.*

Record your thoughts and feelings about specific situations in an anger log. As you build it, you should start to see patterns that give information to better manage similar situations in the future.

Start with three columns. (We'll add additional columns later as we continue through the process.) Label the columns as follows:

- My Pain/Stressors
- What Happened
- What I Thought

At first, you might not be aware of your automatic thoughts, but as you continue to do this exercise, they become more apparent. Start by completing as much as you can each time you feel annoyed, irritated, or angry.

Here's a sample scenario: You and your partner live on a budget and have a rule: Both of you should discuss any purchase over $200 before buying the item. After a trip to the home store for supplies, your partner returns home with $600 worth of outdoor furniture. Any extra money in your budget for the next couple of months is gone, and you didn't have any say in the decision. You are angry because your spouse chose to ignore an agreed-upon household rule and spend a big chunk of your savings without talking to you first.

Your anger log would look like this:

| My Pain/Stressors | What Happened | What I Thought |
| --- | --- | --- |
| It is difficult to save money. | My partner chose to spend money from our savings without talking to me first, even though we previously agreed to discuss purchases over $200 before buying. | My partner should have spoken to me before purchasing the furniture. My partner is inconsiderate. I can't count on my partner to follow household rules. |

Rather than reacting immediately, take a few minutes to complete your anger log. Many times, your emotions change as the situation unfolds, and you want to capture the thoughts that first pop in your head. As you go through the different exercises in this chapter, we will refer to your log and ask you to add to it.

Completing the anger log helps you focus on the thoughts behind your emotions. You can then look for distortions in your thinking and challenge your beliefs.

Review your anger log after a week; look for automatic thoughts based on problematic thought processes and work on finding productive and positive ways to express your feelings.

## Causes of Anger

In Chapter 2, we talked about different types of problematic thought processes. A few of these—intention, blame, and defensiveness—often cause anger.

*Problematic Thought Process:* Intention—you assume a purposeful and harmful intent behind an action.

- Your friend is late for lunch, and you think your friendship isn't important.
- Your spouse doesn't reply to your text, and you assume he or she is angry at you.
- Your boss is in a bad mood, and you assume he isn't happy with your work.

*Counterstrategy:* Depersonalize the act.

Ask yourself, "What are some other reasons that explain the actions of others?"

*New thoughts:*

- Maybe my friend got caught in traffic.
- Maybe my spouse is busy or not looking at her phone right now.
- Maybe he is upset because he didn't sleep well the night before.

*Problematic Thought Process:* Blame—you place the blame on someone else instead of accepting responsibility.

- You blame the taxi driver when you are late for a meeting.
- You blame your coworker for a report being late.
- You blame your spouse for spending too much money.

*Counterstrategy:* Take responsibility.

Ask yourself, "What about this situation is my responsibility?"

*New thoughts:*

- I didn't allow enough time to get across town.
- I didn't get my portion of the report to my coworker on time, which didn't give her enough time to finish.
- I need to look at my spending habits first.

*Problematic Thought Process:* Defensiveness—you believe everything should be done your way and find it difficult to accept there are different ways of doing things.

- Your boss wants you to redo a report to make it more comprehensive. You think, "What a tyrant!"
- Your friend suggests a different route to drive when going out to dinner. You think, "My way would be much faster."

Your spouse chooses a different paint color when deciding what color to paint your living room. You think, "They always criticize my choices."

*Counterstrategy:* Practice empathy.

Ask yourself, "What ideas and experiences does the other person bring to this situation?"

*New thoughts:*

- I see the benefit of the changes my boss requested. They will improve the report and help me improve my work performance.
- I always take the same route; it will be useful to know more than one way to the restaurant.
- Both colors are beautiful. We can get samples and see which one we like on the wall.

When someone criticizes you or makes a complaint, you get to choose how to respond. Your first reaction could be annoyance or defensiveness. Instead, think about what the other person has said. Repeat back what he said to clarify that you understood and are willing to consider his point of view.

At times, you might feel your anger is justified; someone did something wrong, and you have every right to be angry. Suppose you came home from work to find your son playing video games. Before going to work, you left instructions for him to mow the lawn, take out the trash, and clean his room. He did nothing from the list, and even worse, the kitchen is now a mess because he left his breakfast and lunch dishes in the sink. He spent the entire day eating, watching television, and playing video games. You are fuming.

When a situation such as this happens, it is essential to remember that while you can't control the other person's actions, you can manage your response. Sometimes, anger boils up so quickly you feel as if you have no control over it. Remember, you choose your reaction. Before blowing up at your son, take a few minutes to cool down and review the situation. Ask yourself these questions:

- How important will this be in an hour, tomorrow, next week, or next year?
- Is this worth being angry and ruining my entire evening?
- What steps can I take to resolve the situation?

You might decide to turn off the television and video games until he completes the chores. You might decide that you will give your son another chance tomorrow to complete the tasks but make it clear that television and video games are off-limits until he finishes the work. You might take other privileges, such as his cell phone, away until he proves he can follow your instructions. You might decide he needs to text you pictures of the completed chores before he can watch television or play video games.

Listing the choices you have helps you feel in control and reduces the overwhelming feelings of anger. If this doesn't work, remove yourself from the situation by going for a walk, exercising, listening to some music, or enjoying some activity you find relaxing. Once you have calmed down, look at the situation again, and come up with steps to resolve it.

### Your Turn: Criticism, Complaint, or Request?

*The form accompanying this exercise is in Appendix C.*

When someone makes a complaint or request, do you immediately assume she is criticizing what you have done or haven't done? The following exercise helps you look at complaints and requests from both sides—yours and theirs.

| Automatic Thoughts: Criticisms and Complaints | Request and Information Perspective |
| --- | --- |
| He is so demanding. | He is under pressure; the client meeting is on Monday. |
| She doesn't care whether we enjoy our time off. | My boss must think highly of me to ask me to complete this. |
| He isn't happy with my work and wants to punish me. | I do have plans for this evening; maybe I could offer to come in early on Monday to finish this. |
| She is saying the first draft wasn't right. | She didn't say the first draft wasn't any good, just that she wants the final draft completed. |

Instead of jumping to conclusions based on your automatic thoughts, this exercise gives you time to sit down, look at the situation from a different perspective, and find a solution. It helps you to move from anger to problem solving.

## Healthy vs. Unhealthy Anger

Anger itself is neither healthy nor unhealthy. The frequency, intensity, and expression of your anger determine whether it is constructive or destructive. Healthy anger is typically milder, occurs less often, and is used to solve problems and set boundaries for yourself.

Some people have trouble controlling their anger, letting it boil over and explode. They use anger to control, intimidate, manipulate, or punish others. Unhealthy anger is out of proportion to the situation and usually lasts longer than necessary. Unhealthy anger occurs more frequently than healthy anger. Frequent or intense anger is not healthy because it hurts your immune system, increases blood pressure, and sets you up to be angry repeatedly.

The following are unhealthy ways people express anger.

- Yelling
- Screaming
- Fighting
- Blaming
- Threatening
- Violence
- Retaliating
- Holding grudges
- Ending relationships
- Punishing others

Expressing anger in these ways can meet your needs in the short term, but you often end up alienating those around you or creating conflict in your relationships. You might have legal problems because of fights or property destruction. Once you calm down, you might regret what you did or said; even so, when anger strikes again, you still overreact.

Not expressing anger is also unhealthy. You bottle it up inside, never telling anyone how you feel. Suppressed anger is associated with high blood pressure, heart disease, and cancer.

When you manage anger in healthy ways, you use it as a guide to tell you something is wrong. It is your way of noticing disappointment or injustice. Suppose your children are playing outside. A car speeds down the street. You get angry. "What is that car doing? Don't they know children are playing? That is so dangerous!" You have a choice. You can react by running after the car, yelling, and waving your arms, although this probably isn't going to solve anything. You can take affirmative action, getting involved in your community and working with the police to have signs and speed bumps placed on the street. You can use your anger to create change. Expressing anger in this way provides you with a sense of control over your life.

## Your Turn: How Angry Are You?

Review the behaviors on the following chart and think about how often you display them. Rate the frequency and the intensity for each. Use a scale of 0 to 5, with 5 being very frequent or very intense. Add up your score for each column.

| Behavior | Frequency | Intensity |
|---|---|---|
| Yelling | | |
| Screaming | | |
| Verbal fighting | | |
| Physical fighting | | |
| Blaming others | | |
| Making threats | | |
| Acting violently | | |
| Retaliating | | |
| Holding grudges | | |
| Ending relationships | | |
| Punishing others | | |
| Totals | | |

*Total score of 0–22:* You are probably able to manage your anger within reasonable limits. You might still benefit from the skills in this chapter and learn helpful ways of handling frustrating situations.

*Total score of 23–44:* You probably have some anger management problems and need to learn how to manage your reactions differently.

*Total score of 45–55:* It is most likely you have an anger management problem and need to use the skills in this chapter to help you manage your reactions and reach out for help in learning to control anger.

## Common Hot Buttons

Hot buttons are situations that trigger specific attitudes, which in turn, cause anger. While each person has hot buttons specific to his or her life and past experiences, some common themes underlie most people's triggers. You can combat hot button triggers by using coping statements—short declarations that help you manage stressful situations and counterattack triggers. When you practice using these statements, your brain automatically remembers them and creates new mental habits and reflexes.

Let's look at some examples of hot button triggers along with the associated attitudes and some suggested coping statements to help deal with the situation.

*Situation 1:* Things don't go your way.

*Attitude:* You feel entitled to your desires and become annoyed when other people prevent you from getting what you want.

*Coping statements:* "I have wants and needs, but others are entitled to disagree or say no. I need to respect their right to do that," or "I have needs, but others have needs, too."

*Example:* You are up for a promotion at work, but someone else gets it. Instead of thinking, "How dare he; he backstabbed me," practice acceptance. "Everyone at work wants to get ahead. The person who got the promotion deserves it as much as I do."

*Situation 2:* Something is unfair, or someone is taking advantage of you.

*Attitude:* You believe everything should be fair, and if things are not just, you feel the need to correct it.

*Coping Statements:* "I see fairness based on my perspective; other people have their perspectives." "Fairness is subjective. Others have a right to see things according to their ideas, principles, and expectations." "Life is not always fair; that is something I need to accept." "Not every battle is worth fighting."

*Example:* Your friend purchases an expensive necklace. You feel angry and jealous and think, "It's so unfair; I can barely pay my rent." Instead, practice acceptance. "Not everything in life is fair; I'm sure she has her battles, too. It isn't for me to say how she should spend her money."

*Situation 3:* Someone lets you down or doesn't do what you expected.

*Attitude:* You assume others are intentionally trying to harm you or don't care about your needs.

*Coping statements:* "No one is perfect; not everyone behaves the way I would." "When someone doesn't do something that I expect, it doesn't mean they don't care about my needs. Others have their own needs, which might compete with my needs."

*Example:* Your partner forgets your birthday, and you assume it means he doesn't care enough to remember or is intentionally trying to hurt your feelings. Instead, think: "I accept he is not good about remembering social events. I can remind him my birthday is approaching rather than setting him up to feel guilty."

*Situation 4:* Others around you make the same mistakes repeatedly.

*Attitude:* You believe that you need to change them. You think if you try hard enough, yell, or complain enough, you will eventually whip them into shape.

*Coping statement:* "Other people have their methods and limits. Demanding they change without understanding their motivations and limitations only leads to dead ends."

*Example:* Your employee keeps handing in reports in an incoherent manner. You think, "What an incompetent idiot; why is he so defiant?" Instead, try thinking, "Apparently, he does not understand what I want in this report. I will set up a time for us to go over exactly how to complete these reports."

Think about a recent situation that made you upset. Write down a short description of the events. Ask yourself: What can I do to change my perception of what happened? Then write a coping statement.

# Reframe Your Emotion

Some of the most common problematic thinking processes in anger are personalization and labeling. When you label situations, others, or yourself using extreme language, you escalate your anger and mood. Behaviors such as cursing, name-calling, or exaggerating the negativity ("This is awful!" "No one ever treated me so poorly!") make the situation worse rather than better. Instead of living in disbelief, try to accept what transpired.

When going through a challenging situation, keep track of the descriptive words you use. Replace the terms with more objective or moderate descriptions. Then, repeat your original statement using the new words and see if the level of intensity of your emotion decreases.

*Original statement:* "I can't believe he forgot my birthday! I am furious!"

*New statement:* "He forgot my birthday. This is disappointing. I'm annoyed."

*Original statement:* "I can't believe FedEx lost my package! These drivers are idiots. What a disaster. I am so upset. I need to report him."

*New statement:* "FedEx lost my package. This is frustrating. I need to call and file a claim."

# Accept Fallibility in Yourself and Others

You know you are not a perfect person. You know you make mistakes, and you know you have faults—you just prefer not to think about them. After all, when you think about your weaknesses, you must either accept you are wrong, or you must commit to change. Ignoring your faults is much more comfortable. But, you expect others to see and take responsibility for their flaws and mistakes; when they don't, you get angry.

Disarming anger begins with accepting that everyone, including yourself, is fallible. Once you do, it is easier to see your anger triggers from a different perspective. Suppose your partner forgets your birthday. You are angry because they didn't live up to your expectations. You assume he is inconsiderate. However, if you see your partner as fallible, then the situation and your perception of it changes. "He is forgetful, but he expresses love in other ways. I forgot things before and hoped people understood. I should understand when he is forgetful."

You might become angry when people do not behave the way you think they should and judge them based on how you perceive their actions. For example, suppose you are talking to a coworker when another coworker comes along and interrupts the conversation. You think he is rude. What your attitude implies is "He should behave the way I would." If you judge yourself first, remembering that you have interrupted others in the past or have done things others believed was wrong or inappropriate, then you are more apt to view other people's behavior differently. Remember, it is not your responsibility to change other people. It is your responsibility to monitor and adjust your responses and reactions.

Another way to minimize judging others is when you notice it, stop, and immediately find one thing you like about the other person. Praise him or her for that quality. Doing so makes you stop and see the person differently.

## Your Turn: Judge Yourself First

Try to catch yourself labeling someone. Pay attention and listen to how often you judge others—sometimes, kindly, and other times, not so much. Whenever you negatively judge someone, stop, and label your behavior first. For example, when a coworker interrupts your conversation, you might be impatient or intolerant. When you name your actions, you can focus on changing them rather than expecting someone else to change.

## Increase Your Frustration Tolerance

Do you get annoyed over little details? Do you find yourself irritated whenever something goes wrong? You might have what is called low frustration tolerance. Typical problematic thought processes include catastrophizing or overgeneralizing about your frustration. You think being frustrated is terrible, so you avoid any type of disappointment. You deny yourself practice in coping with frustration.

When you have a low frustration tolerance, you demand everything be the way you want it to be. You don't see levels of problems; there is no such thing as a "small" problem. You see everything as a catastrophe. When you have a low frustration tolerance, you…

- Seek activities that give immediate pleasure.
- Spend your time trying to avoid pain.
- Complain.
- Become distressed over small setbacks.

- Are overly concerned about fairness.
- Tend to compare your circumstances to other people's circumstances.

People with low frustration tolerance have a higher risk of addiction or impulsive behaviors such as unsafe sex or overspending. They tend to have a "short fuse," quickly angering when things go wrong.

When frustrated about a specific problem, write about it. Use one of the following viewpoints to see the situation from different perspectives:

- Write a letter to your best friend describing what happened and the steps you plan to take to improve it.
- Imagine you are alone on a desert island. Write a letter describing the situation and how your life improved once you solved it. You are going to put it into a bottle and throw it into the sea for a potential rescuer to read.
- Write a letter to yourself from the future. View the situation from 1 month, 1 year, and 3 years from now. Describe the situation and how you resolved it.
- Write a worst-case scenario describing the absolute worst that could happen. Think about the physical and emotional problems that might ensue if the problem continues. Imagine life after the worst possible solution occurs.

Once you look at the problem from different perspectives, it often doesn't seem as bad as it initially did.

## Your Turn: Raise Your Frustration Tolerance

You can use the ABCDEF chart to analyze your frustration and come up with ways to change your reaction.

**A:** Activating Event

**B:** Beliefs

**C:** Consequences

**D:** Problematic Thinking Processes

**E:** New Thoughts

**F:** Coping Statement

Let's look at an example.

**A:** My supervisor criticized me in front of my coworkers.

**B:** It was very unfair. She should have spoken to me in private instead of treating me like a child. It was humiliating; everyone looked at me. I can't deal with someone treating me without respect.

**C:** I was angry for the rest of the day. I couldn't concentrate and didn't get much work done. I want to quit.

**D:** Personalization and blame, "should" and "must," and emotional reasoning.

**E:** I would have preferred that my supervisor had spoken with me in private, but she doesn't need to do things the way I want. It would be better if she treated me with respect, but sometimes that isn't going to happen. I was uncomfortable and embarrassed, but it was not the worst thing that has ever happened to me. I am sure no one is judging me; after all, other people get reprimanded at work, and I don't judge them.

**F:** I would prefer it if I did not carry anger with me all day when things don't go as I think they should. I would prefer to view negative situations differently and remember I have survived worse.

When thinking about your desired behavior or reaction, avoid replacing an intensely negative emotion with a profoundly positive feeling. Instead, work on moving to a more moderate response. Use the emotion levels and other words described in Chapter 4. For example, instead of "furious," try "annoyed."

Anger is neither good nor bad. The frequency, intensity, and how you express it determines if it is positive or destructive. Unhealthy anger sometimes offers short-term benefits, but in the long term, it can create problems in your relationships and at work, as well as decrease satisfaction with life. You choose how to respond; rewording your thoughts can change your perspective.

# CHAPTER 19
# Managing OCD

You think you forgot to turn off the stove and you go back to check it—sometimes four or five times. Before leaving the house, you systematically check every window and door to assure yourself they are locked. You spend hours organizing and reorganizing your bookshelves, placing books alphabetically or by color. We all have daily routines. They keep us focused and improve productivity. But if you have obsessive-compulsive disorder (OCD), your habits and behaviors become obsessions and compulsions that take up time and interfere with daily life. This chapter helps you understand the relationship between obsessions and compulsions and provides strategies to help lessen your dependence on rituals.

## Understanding Obsessive-Compulsive Disorder

Obsessive-compulsive disorder (OCD) is an anxiety disorder characterized by obsessions and compulsions. Obsessions are intrusive and upsetting thoughts, images, or impulses that repeatedly occur in your mind. Compulsions are thoughts, behaviors, and/or rituals you use to reduce the obsessions. Compulsions are often repeated and done to relieve obsessive thoughts. You feel powerless to control both. It is a spectrum disorder, meaning it ranges from mild to severe.

For example, suppose you worry about germs; you are afraid when you touch someone or something, you will become ill. These thoughts overtake you, and you must wash your hands, sometimes hundreds of times a day. Until you do, you can't focus and are agitated. In more severe cases of OCD, you have a ritual, such as washing your hands five times. You perform this ritual to try to diminish the thoughts about germs; however, it probably only provides short-term relief. Often, rituals accompany obsessions, but that isn't always true. They can be mental without a physical component.

Obsessions and rituals vary from person to person; however, there are frequently common themes:

- Distressing religious or sacrilegious thoughts; for example, ideas about joining a cult or worrying about religious persecution for your sins.
- Intrusive thoughts of violent acts, such as having hurt someone in the past or harming someone in the future.
- Sexual thoughts or images; for example, worrying you have a sexually transmitted disease, that you did something inappropriate, or worrying that you are gay when you are straight or vice versa.
- Constant worry about contamination from dirt, germs, bodily fluids, and other materials.
- Worry about throwing away something essential or needing something you threw away; for example, hoarding newspapers, communications, tax papers, or clothing.
- Constant worry that you made a mistake or that you will make a mistake.
- Worry that you have a disease, focusing on a real or imagined symptom, and concern that you are dying.

Common rituals:

- Spending excessive time organizing things to make them "right," such as lining things up, arranging items by color or alphabetically, making lists, or reorganizing files.
- Washing hands, kitchen counters, and bathrooms excessively.
- Repeatedly checking to make sure you completed a task; for example, turning off the oven, locking the door, or rereading communication.
- Repeating words or phrases, such as repeating a specific word 10 times before starting a task.
- Self-assurances, such as talking yourself out the obsession: "It will be okay; nothing is going to happen."
- Asking others for reassurance.
- Mental rituals to replace bad thoughts or images with good thoughts or images.
- Counting.
- Repeating a phrase a certain number of times.
- Seeking reassurance or medical advice; for example, surfing the internet for medical diagnoses or repeatedly checking with friends and family to make sure things will turn out okay.

When you live with OCD, you might become irritated or distressed when interrupted or prevented from performing rituals. You might seek constant reassurance from your partner, friends, or family, asking for assurance that nothing bad will occur, you don't have a disease, or your appearance is acceptable. Some people who have obsessive thoughts about doing a violent act might believe they are terrible or evil.

When you try to avoid obsessive thoughts or resist completing compulsions, it seems unbearable. Your obsessions and compulsions take time out of your day; sometimes, you spend several hours each day replaying obsessive thoughts or performing rituals. Rituals are not always external or physical acts; they are occasionally internal, such as counting, going through a checklist in your mind, or creating an elaborate plan to overcome a disaster.

Many people who experience obsessions recognize that their beliefs are untrue, and the need to complete their ritual is simply a way to alleviate their anxiety. Even so, they feel powerless to stop. Other times, the obsession could be accurate, but the intensity, frequency, and duration of the fear or anxiety, and the lengths to stop thinking about it, that creates an issue.

# Your Turn: Identify Your Triggers

Keep a log for several days to discover possible triggers for your obsessive thoughts. If you experience many obsessive thoughts each day, just note 3 to 5 per day instead of noting every obsession.

| Trigger | Obsession | Compulsion |
| --- | --- | --- |
| Took out trash | Germs on trash | Washed hands with soap five times |
| Loaned someone a pen | Germs from the other person on the pen | Threw out pen |
| Used a shopping cart | Germs on the cart from other people | Wore latex gloves while shopping |

This example includes obsessions about germs; your obsession might be different, or you might note various obsessions.

Keep in mind the world is ever changing. For example, during the COVID-19 pandemic, most people became more aware of germs, washing shopping carts before using them, using hand sanitizer throughout the day, and avoiding sharing items. Suddenly, it wasn't a problem to be constantly worried about germs and infections. But it is possible that people with OCD found this time even more difficult and overwhelming. If worry about germs interferes with your daily functioning, even during a pandemic, it is problematic.

Make a list of several of your obsessions; choose one to start with, and think about your triggers. You can use the ladder technique, described in the exercise "Ladder Rungs" in Chapter 5, listing your triggers in order from easiest to hardest. Begin by working on the most comfortable trigger first, and work your way up the ladder.

## Thoughts Are Just Thoughts

It is impossible to avoid your thoughts; they run through your mind even when you are not conscious of them. In CBT therapy for OCD, the goal is not necessarily to challenge your thoughts, but rather learn to accept that feelings are there without attaching any validity and meaning to them. When you attempt to resolve an irrational belief with a rational one, you could inadvertently use that as a ritual going forward. For example, if your irrational thought is, "I might get sick from touching the shopping cart," replacing it with a rational thought can quickly become a ritual—you feel you must say it before touching a shopping cart.

A thought is just a thought; when you connect a purpose, you react to it and are more likely to continue having it.

## Your Turn: Thought Exposure

When using exposure therapy, you physically face your fears, but when you have OCD, you are frequently facing obsessive thoughts. This type of exposure therapy involves writing down your obsessive thoughts in detail.

Start by writing down your obsessive thoughts. Fill in as many details as you can. Write down how you feel, what you want to do, and how strong your urge to complete a ritual or compulsion is.

For the next 2 weeks, write a description of the same obsessive thought. It might change slightly, but the focus should remain the same. Writing your obsessions could trigger new obsessions, or you might create additional scenarios revolving around the same obsession. Don't worry; this is normal. Keep writing about it every day. This exercise works to desensitize you to your obsession.

## Overcoming Magical Thinking

Magical thinking is when you believe that if you do something or don't do something, it affects your environment or the world. For example, you might think completing a specific good-bye ritual with your children each morning keeps them safe throughout the day. Many people with OCD experience these types of thoughts, reinforcing their need to act on their compulsions.

Gathering evidence to disprove your obsession is one way to combat magical thinking. The following is an example of how this works.

*Obsession:* I worry that my house will burn down because I forgot to turn the stove off.

*Compulsion:* I need to check the stove five times before leaving the house.

*Magical thinking:* If I do not check the stove five times, it will be my fault if something bad happens.

*Gathering evidence:* Think back to a time you did not check the stove five times. Did your house burn down? Did something bad happen at your house? Did your prediction come true?

Practice by delaying the completion of your ritual. Challenge your belief that something is going to happen (or not happen) as a direct result of your compulsions.

When you work to reduce compulsions, it is vital to postpone completing your ritual without looking for evidence or challenging the thought. Performing the ritual is considered a mental form of seeking reassurance.

## Response Prevention

When you delay performing a routine, it is uncomfortable. You use compulsive behavior to avoid feeling discomfort. It is supposed to relieve your anxiety. When you delay completing the ritual, you might feel agitated, irritable, or unfocused, but this is a crucial step in reducing your need for your compulsive behaviors. Delaying or ignoring your urge to complete a ritual and lessening your dependence on completing rituals is called *response prevention*.

Response prevention works like this: You have a cold and start obsessing. What if it is more dangerous? What if it means you have a severe disease? What if you are going to die? To relieve health obsessions, you usually surf the internet. You research your symptoms, looking for reassurance that you aren't deathly ill—that is your ritual. The first step is to wait 15 minutes before giving in to your desire to search the web. When 15 minutes has passed, if you still have the urge to carry out the ritual, ask yourself, "Can I handle the discomfort for another 15 minutes?" Try to delay the ritual another 15 minutes. In the beginning, you might find it very difficult not to give in to the routine. Eventually, it becomes more comfortable; the more you resist your compulsion, the more your obsession subsides.

## Behavioral Experiments

In Chapter 10, you learned to create a new belief and test its validity. This technique is helpful when trying to change obsessive thoughts.

*Situation:* When getting ready to leave the house, you walk around and check to see if every door and window is locked. When done, you do it a second time.

*Belief:* I must check all the doors and windows twice before I leave the house to keep it safe.

*Experiment:* I will leave the house for 15 minutes after checking the doors and windows once.

You check the doors and windows and leave the house, despite the strong urges to check again. Your heart is racing, and you feel shaky. You take a walk for 15 minutes; you can't stop worrying that something terrible is happening at your house. After 15 minutes, you return home to find that nothing awful has occurred. The house is the same as when you left. You complete this experiment several times and have similar results. You slowly start to increase the time you are away from the house.

Let's look at another example.

*Situation:* You have a fear of getting sick from drinking from a public water fountain. You always carry water to avoid using a water fountain. You become agitated if your children ask to get a drink from a water fountain.

*Belief:* My children or I will get sick if we use a water fountain.

*Experiment:* Drink from the water fountain.

You go to the mall and take a drink from the water fountain. For the next few days, you are hypervigilant. Do you have a fever? Is your throat scratchy? But nothing happens. You don't get sick. You repeat the experiment several times over the next couple of weeks, using different water fountains. You still don't get sick. Your obsession slowly starts to disappear.

When creating a behavior experiment, decide how you are going to know whether your prediction comes true. Vague statements such as "to see what happens" won't give you information to disprove your original belief. Specific statements, such as "If no one gets sick within 3 days of drinking a water fountain," work best.

To reap the benefits of behavioral experiments, you should repeat the same test several times. Each time reinforces your new belief. When you master one compulsion, where you feel no anxiety, move on to another experiment.

# Exposure Therapy

We discussed exposure therapy for specific fears in Chapter 17. The same technique can help relieve your anxiety about certain situations when you have OCD.

Start by making a list of actions that provoke your intrusive thoughts or compulsions, such as shaking someone's hand. The more you confront the fear and learn nothing happens, the less control your fear has over you. The anxiety surrounding shaking someone's hand should slowly diminish.

Rank situations on your list from mild to severe, with those that cause only mild stress on the bottom of your list. Begin your exposure exercises with these and work your way up your list to those that cause more significant anxiety. Stay with each situation until you feel comfortable, and your need to perform your routine lessens.

Begin your exposure gradually. Using the example of shaking a person's hand, start with friends or relatives. Work your way up to shaking a stranger's hand. It is crucial to resist your urge to perform any rituals after exposure. Your rituals reinforce your fears; therefore, you can't move past those fears without stopping your routine.

Keep track of your anxiety level. In the beginning, you might rate it at 100 percent, but as you practice, your rating should decrease. You can use this technique in conjunction with behavioral experiments, noting in your log that you did not get sick after shaking someone's hand. Use the rating and information in your record to reevaluate your beliefs and challenge their validity.

Sometimes, you can't face your perceived fears because they are not an object or situation. Suppose you check your stove repeatedly to relieve the anxiety your house is going to burn down. You can't face the fear of your home burning down. Instead, use imagery; create detailed images of the disaster you fear could happen. In this example, you would imagine your house burning down and resist the urge to check the stove.

# Tips for Reducing Rituals

By working on changing your thinking, you can reduce the obsessions and your need for rituals. The following are tips to help you.

*Manage stress.* Stress is often a trigger for OCD symptoms. Create a plan to deal with stress. Chapter 15 goes over strategies to use in everyday life to reduce stress. The relaxation techniques in Chapter 7 are also helpful. One quick tip is to take 10 slow, deep breaths when in a stressful situation.

*Be flexible.* When you have obsessions, you usually catastrophize. You believe disasters will occur if you don't do a particular ritual or worry about contracting a significant illness or disease. You think you or a family member might be involved in a horrible car crash. No matter what your thoughts, the outcome is usually horrific. This type of thinking can boil over to other parts of your life. You might be overprotective of your children, anxious every time your significant other leaves the house, or have excessive absences at work because you are obsessed with illness. If these sound like you, reread Chapter 12 to learn strategies to lower your inner criticism and eliminate your need to have everything in your life turn out perfectly.

Live with uncertainty. Uncertainty is a part of life. If you have OCD, not knowing what to expect or not being able to control your environment is probably challenging. You perform rituals to control events in the future. Stopping your routines doesn't guarantee that nothing wrong is going to happen. But there isn't a guarantee that it isn't going to happen, even when you do complete your rituals. In Chapter 17, you learn strategies for accepting that life is full of uncertainty and managing fears of an unknown future.

Let go of internal measurement. If you have OCD, you might measure when to stop checking the stove as when you feel "comfortable." You might stop washing your hands when it feels "right." These measurements are based on internal feelings, not on facts or external measures. Use specific measurements for your obsessions, such as "washing my hands with soap and water for thirty seconds is enough."

Don't give thoughts too much weight. If you have OCD, you probably disregard facts and attach importance to your ideas. For example, if you have a cold, you ignore the fact that your symptoms indicate you have a cold. Instead, you focus on your thoughts, which tell you that this is a sign of a significant illness. Remind yourself that thoughts are just thoughts. Focus on the facts.

## Build on Successes

Every time you manage to delay or eliminate performing a ritual, you make progress. Good job! Some days you might not feel like you are making any progress, and it is good to remember these successes. Keep a log of every success, no matter how small. Reminding yourself of your accomplishments motivates you to continue.

Managing your OCD takes practice. Commit to using the skills in this chapter every day. Over time, your fears and anxieties will no longer have control over you. Consistency is the key to learning how to manage your OCD. If you do not feel happy with your level of progression in managing your OCD, seek the help of a doctor or therapist.

Setbacks are normal. There could be times when a fear resurfaces; one you thought you conquered reappears suddenly. Don't worry. Look back over your exercises, see what worked, and start again. It isn't going to take as long as it did the first time, especially if you catch the fear immediately. For example, suppose you worked on not washing your hands after touching something. You were doing great, and a few weeks later, you started having urges to wash your hands repeatedly. Refocus your attention and touch the object without washing your hands for 5 minutes.

Remember, anxiety usually lessens on its own. Distress rises in intensity, peaks, and then decreases. Sometimes, you simply need to wait it out and give your fear a chance to subside.

Obsessions are intrusive and upsetting thoughts; compulsions are rituals—physical or mental—you complete to relieve the stress they cause. Sometimes, you use magical thinking, believing your routines influence external events. Reducing the need for rituals is hard work and causes discomfort in the short term but benefits you in the long term.

# CHAPTER 20
# Developing a Positive Body Image

You watch what you eat, check the scale every morning, and skip meals if you gained even a pound. When you look in the mirror, you see everything you perceive as wrong, a nose that is too big, a forehead that is too long, and hair that is too thick, too thin, or disappearing. Or you might avoid looking in the mirror because you find your appearance distressing. You focus on what you perceive as wrong and believe that when other people look at you, they also see all the faults and negatively judge you for them. In this chapter, you learn what it means to have a poor body image and how problematic thought processes contribute to it. The exercises help you define yourself by character traits rather than appearance.

## What Is Body Image?

Body image is how you think and feel about your body. It is a combination of the picture in your mind, the image in the mirror, your feelings about those images, and how you think you compare to others. Everyone has parts of their bodies they would like to change. You might think your nose is too big or your chin too pointy. You might wish your hips were a little smaller or your thighs thinner. When you believe your faults reflect your self-worth, you probably have a body image problem.

## Healthy vs. Unhealthy Body Image

When you have a healthy body image, you accept how you look. You might not believe you are perfect, but you recognize your positive traits and your flaws. Even when you work to change those flaws, you accept your appearance and don't allow it to color your opinion of yourself. You don't dwell on people who don't see you as attractive. You believe that someone could be or is attracted to you physically, and your appearance is only one part of your whole self.

An unhealthy body image places too much emphasis on appearance. You equate a large part of your value as a person to your looks. You are so unhappy with your weight, your size, your shape, or other attributes that it keeps you from enjoying social encounters or accepting compliments. You are embarrassed in public and often spend hours hiding or disguising your body or avoiding going outside at all.

## Your Turn: Do You Have a Body Image Problem?

Check off any of the following statements that are relevant to you:

- ❏ I am unhappy with my looks or how a body part looks despite reassurance from others.
- ❏ Sometimes I don't go out socially because of my appearance.
- ❏ I spend a considerable amount of time daily thinking about or worrying about my appearance.
- ❏ I spend considerable time trying to find clothing that hides my imperfections.
- ❏ I avoid clothes shopping because I am not happy with how I look.
- ❏ At times, I avoid looking at myself in the mirror or repeatedly check my appearance.
- ❏ I make excuses to avoid situations, such as going to the beach or the pool, where I need to have my body exposed.
- ❏ I believe physical appearance is extremely important. I think others judge me solely based on physical appearance.
- ❏ I often compare how I look to other's appearances. If I don't feel as attractive as someone else, I get upset.
- ❏ I avoid intimate relationships or sexual situations because I don't feel comfortable with someone seeing or touching my body.
- ❏ I consistently diet or look for ways to improve my physical appearance.
- ❏ I feel driven to work out, to lose weight, or improve my body shape. I feel guilty if I skip one exercise routine or miss a day of exercise.
- ❏ I don't believe other people when they say I look nice.
- ❏ If someone doesn't like me, I think it's because I'm ugly.
- ❏ I use or research cosmetic surgery or other dermatological treatments to correct flaws in my appearance.

If you checked five or more items, you could have a problem with body image. The exercises in this chapter can help resolve these issues; however, if your body image problem is severe, you might consider working with a therapist.

To start combatting an unhealthy body image, write a list of 10 things you like about yourself that don't have anything to do with your weight or appearance. Your list could include "good friend," "hard worker," or "good at decorating." Keep this list in a place where you see it regularly.

## Problematic Thinking Processes

In Chapter 2, you learned about problematic thinking processes. People with body image problems might use the following processes:

*Overgeneralizing:* You see flaws in your appearance as proof of "I am not worthy" and assume "Others think I am unattractive because of this flaw." You believe you can't change. For example, if dieting was unsuccessful in the past, you assume it always will be, or if someone does not find you attractive, you believe no one will ever think you are appealing.

*Magnification:* You obsess and magnify the importance of one part of your body. For example, if you have a pimple, you think it ruins your entire appearance and that no one can see past it. If you put on a few pounds, you see yourself as "fat." You define your entire appearance around one body part or issue.

*Black-and-white thinking:* You compare yourself to everyone and categorize yourself and others as either "attractive" or "not attractive." You don't consider the gray areas in your attractiveness or your behaviors. For example, you categorize eating habits as either, "I am on a diet" or "I am overindulging," rather than focusing on healthy eating habits. You see yourself as either a "slob" or "perfectly put together."

*Ignoring the positive:* You discount compliments you receive based on your appearance. You don't believe it when others compliment you; you assume they are just being nice or devalue their importance. For example, if someone says, "You look great; you've lost weight!" you think they are pointing out that you have more weight to lose.

*Mind reading:* You assume that others judge you because of your looks. You believe everyone thinks you are fat, ugly, have a big nose, and so on.

*Personalization and blame:* You avoid taking responsibility for your interactions. For example, you might think, "He didn't like me because I am overweight," rather than "We didn't have a lot in common" and blame any rejection on your looks. You call yourself names like "fat," "ugly," and "disgusting" instead of thinking objectively: "I am 20 pounds heavier than I would like to be."

*Fortune-telling:* You decide how the future is going to turn out and think, "No one will ever want to go out with me because of my big nose," or "I will never stay on a diet." When you are rejected or go off your diet, you feel validated in your predictions.

# Your Turn: Changing the Image

"Fat talk," is often considered harmless. This is the banter among women about their bodies, such as "My thighs look so big in these jeans," "I feel fat today," or "This ice cream is going straight to my hips." But one study found that women who use this type of talk regularly are more unhappy with their bodies than those who don't and may have a higher risk of eating disorders.

Use a chart to record negative thoughts about your body in different situations. Then restructure your thoughts about yourself and your body.

| Negative Statements | Problematic Thought Processes | New Thoughts |
|---|---|---|
| I am fat. She is skinny. | Black-and-white thinking | I weigh about 15 pounds more than she does; this does not mean I am obese or that no one thinks I am attractive. |
| I had a bite of my spouse's burger and fries, so I am off my diet. I should have a dessert and start again tomorrow. | Black-and-white thinking | Developing healthy eating habits is much more important than following a diet. |
| I am short. Women like tall men. | Magnification | I cannot change my height, but I am a good person and am loyal and loving. I will find the right person. |

# How Body Image Affects Your Life

People with body image problems magnify the significance of flaws and ignore how much their flaws limit or don't limit their life. For example, you are very self-conscious about your large ears. But you are successful and satisfied with your professional and personal life. Your perceived large ears haven't interfered with your life. Think about how much your concern with your body image limits your life. Let's look at some examples.

*Scenario 1:* You see someone thinner than you.

*Unhealthy thought:* I am so fat; why can't I lose weight and look like her? I am going to skip dinner tonight.

*Acceptance thought:* She is thinner than me, but I am happy with my appearance.

*Scenario 2:* While getting dressed in the morning, you look in the mirror and notice your hair is thinning.

*Unhealthy thought:* I am going bald. Everyone will notice.

*Acceptance thought:* I don't have as much hair as I used to, but many men have thinning hair, and it doesn't stop them from enjoying their lives.

*Scenario 3:* You joined a dating app and haven't gotten any dates, matches, or even interest from someone.

*Unhealthy thought:* Everyone is turned off by my looks. I will never get a date.

*Acceptance thought:* I should research the best way to write a profile for these types of apps, so others will be more apt to see mine. I should look through the profiles and express my interest in other people.

*Scenario 4:* You think your nose is too big.

*Unhealthy thought:* My nose is too big; I can't stop thinking about it. When I speak to people, I am sure they are staring at my nose.

*Acceptance thought:* I wish my nose were smaller, but it is not. I have other positive physical traits.

Everyone has flaws, some minor and some major. Everyone also has strengths and positive qualities. When you accept your imperfections, you can move past them, without giving up on improving yourself. For example, if you are overweight, you can acknowledge where you are now and take steps to make healthy changes. You can accept that being overweight doesn't define who you are as a person, but it also does not stop you from making healthy eating choices.

# Your Turn: The Real Impact

*The form accompanying this exercise is in Appendix C.*

This exercise helps you see your flaws and evaluate how much they influence your life.

*Step 1:* Write down what you believe to be a significant flaw in your appearance.

*Step 2:* Write down how this flaw limits your life. Make a list of all your concerns.

*Step 3:* Find evidence to counter your assumptions and create a coping statement.

Let's look at an example.

*Step 1:* I am overweight.

*Step 2:* Being overweight limits me in these ways:

- No one will think I am attractive.
- People will make fun of me; no one will like me.
- People will stare, so I need to avoid talking to them.

*Step 3:* Counter evidence and coping statement

*Counter evidence:* The last time I went to a social outing and talked to people, I did okay. I met some new people and made new friends.

*Coping statement:* When I put myself out there, I can positively connect with others.

*Counter evidence:* I have friends.

*Coping statement:* I can connect with others. Not everyone wants to avoid me.

*Counter evidence:* No one has laughed at me or pointed out my weight since I was a teenager. People usually act like respectful adults.

*Coping statement:* This social event will be a safe place; the hosts want me to be there.

Finally, make a list of 10 people you admire. Your list might include musicians, artists, a person in your community, a colleague, a teacher at your child's school, or a neighbor who is always willing to help others. Chances are the people on your list have different shapes. Some might wear glasses; some might be bald; others might have big noses. You probably didn't list these people for their appearances; you admire them because of their behaviors and personalities. Remember, just as you don't judge people by how they look, they don't judge you that way.

# Standing in Your Way

Your behavior can perpetuate your fears and reinforce your belief that you should hide your body or specific parts of your body from others. Look through the following behaviors and determine which ones you use. There are suggestions to help you change your actions.

*Avoidance:* You might avoid shopping for clothes, going to the beach or pool, posting pictures and selfies online, or participating in activities where you expose your body. You might avoid intimate relationships. You might avoid social situations because you are afraid others judge you. You might avoid going out of your house unless necessary. Avoidance works in the short term—you feel better because you avoid being uncomfortable. In the long term, however, avoidance can cause loneliness and depression. You don't give yourself the chance to learn that others aren't judging you by your appearance. You don't allow yourself to believe that you can cope with the situation and that appearance doesn't matter as much as you think it does.

Use exposure strategies, as described in Chapter 17. Intentionally act in ways that disprove your beliefs, such as not wearing a hat to cover your bald spot, going out in flats instead of heels if you are self-conscious about being short. Pay attention to whether other people react by pointing, staring, or treating you disrespectfully. If they don't, it should reinforce that your appearance doesn't influence how others treat you.

*Body Checking:* You need to weigh yourself several times a day. You need to look at yourself in the mirror for extended periods to see how you look or check to see if your camouflage worked. Body checking focuses on the worst parts of your appearance and reinforces fears. You are preoccupied with not being good enough. You focus on your feelings about your body, not how you look.

Stand in front of a full-length mirror. Describe your body as if you were describing it to someone over the phone. Don't add in any judgments, just the facts. Don't skip over parts you don't like. This exercise helps you see your body more objectively without evaluating it. Repeat this exercise until you no longer feel anxious.

Or avoid checking your appearance altogether. Initially, the anxiety builds, but eventually, it subsides. Each day, the unease and urge to check will lessen. Then slowly introduce looking in the mirror or weighing yourself on a scheduled basis, such as getting on the scale once a week or looking in the mirror only when dressing and grooming.

*Misinterpreting external signals:* You interpret everyday events or things as evidence that others perceive you are ugly or fat. For example, you go on a date, and the other person is not interested in a second date. You assume it's because you are not attractive. You personalize rejection.

Consider alternative reasons for rejection when dating, not getting a job, or other times you believe others do not want your presence. Using the example of someone not wanting a second date, you could write: We did not have much in common, our interests and ideas were very different.

# See Yourself as a Whole Person

When you receive a gift, you notice the packaging. It could be small or big. The wrapping might be colorful.

It might have a bow. The wrapping might look beautiful or look hastily wrapped. But what is important is the gift inside. Your body is the same. Your body is the packaging; it is what contains who you are. When you focus on your body, you tend to lose sight of the essential things. You view the package as more important than the gift inside.

Complete a whole-person review to remind yourself about your internal traits. Write down as many points as you can in each of the following categories:

- Values—what are the philosophies you use in your life?
- Hobbies and interests—what do you enjoy doing in your spare time?
- Talents and skills—what do you see as your talent? What skills have you learned to help you at school, work, or at home?
- Personality traits—how do you see yourself?

- Spiritual beliefs—what do you believe about God or the universe? What do you see as your purpose in life?
- Humor—what makes you laugh?
- Future goals—where do you see yourself in 10 years? What are some things you would like to accomplish in life?

Write down as many answers as possible, except any that relate to your appearance. Think about qualities you consider important in other people. Is your opinion about other people based on their appearance, or is it based on internal traits?

Create a pie chart of your "whole self." Place all the things you think are included in your personality, such as a good friend, creativity, and a good listener. How much of the pie did you attribute to appearance? Remind yourself each day that how you look is only one part of who you are. Focus on the other areas by spending more time and energy in the next two weeks on these traits. For example, if you put being a good friend at 10 percent, instead of spending 20 minutes in the morning checking your appearance, spend 20 minutes calling, texting, or emailing friends to check in and wish them a great day.

# A Word About Eating Disorders

A poor body image doesn't mean you have an eating disorder; however, there are some features common to both, such as preoccupation with appearance. If you have an eating disorder, you worry about your weight and body shape and are preoccupied with food. When you have a body image problem, you might worry about these things, but you obsess about your overall appearance or one body part.

An eating disorder is a mental illness that causes disturbances in eating patterns. It can involve undereating or overeating. Obsessions about food can take over your life. You are overly concerned about body weight and body shape.

There are three main types of eating disorders:

*Anorexia nervosa* This disorder is characterized by an unhealthy effort to maintain a weight far below the norm for your age and height. People who suffer from anorexia starve themselves or eat very little to prevent weight gain or to continue losing weight. They might also feel driven to exercise excessively.

*Bulimia nervosa* This disorder is characterized by a cycle of overeating and then purging to alleviate feelings of guilt and shame from the overeating. Purging includes self-induced vomiting, overexercise, or the use of laxatives.

*Binge-eating disorder* This disorder is characterized by a compulsive need to eat large amounts of food in a short period. People who binge eat often feel they have no control over their eating and are commonly overweight.

Eating disorders cause serious health issues. If you or someone you know shows the signs of an eating disorder, contact a medical professional. While CBT could be a part of the treatment for eating disorders, it is crucial to involve medical professionals.

When you have a healthy body image, you accept that you can have flaws in your appearance but that these flaws do not define who you are as a person. Some problematic thinking processes commonly associated with poor body image include overgeneralization and mind reading. Many people believe their flaws limit parts of their lives, such as relationships and work; however, it is your perception of these flaws that cause limitations, not the imperfections themselves. Poor body image and eating disorders have some characteristics in common, but they are separate problems.

# CHAPTER 21
# CBT for Grief

Grief is a feeling of deep sorrow for something or someone you lost. We usually equate it with the death of a loved one; however, you can grieve other losses, such as the loss of a marriage, a career, or health. In this chapter, we address grief resulting from death, but you can use the concepts and exercises with other losses.

## What Is Grief?

Grief does not exist in a single moment, and there isn't a time limit for how long someone takes to go through the process of mourning. It encompasses our emotional, physical, and spiritual methods of coping with a loss.

In the book *On Death and Dying*, author Elisabeth Kubler Ross identifies five stages of grief: denial, anger, bargaining, depression, and acceptance. These provide a framework for understanding the intense feelings we have when a loved one dies; however, these feelings aren't universal. Some people skip steps, and others experience them in a different order, jump between stages, or spend years in one step. Everyone experiences and shows grief differently. Your relationship with the deceased, the circumstances around their death, and your life experiences influence how you feel and express sorrow.

There are also different styles of grieving. One person could find that talking about their loved one provides comfort; others might avoid speaking about them for a time. Some might keep themselves busy, and others might become withdrawn. There is no right or wrong way to grieve, and our sorrow is not a reflection of our feelings for the deceased.

Different religions and cultures have customs regarding mourning, the public display of grief—for example, wearing black for a set amount of time after the death. Your relationship with the deceased often determines the mourning period. For example, mourning for a spouse or child is usually more prolonged than for a sibling. But grief doesn't follow a timetable. You might feel the intense pain of loss for days, weeks, months, or years. Usually, it is most intense shortly after death with feelings of sadness lessening over time as you learn to live without the deceased's presence. No matter how much time has passed, triggers, such as mementos, can cause the grief to come crashing down on you.

Grief encompasses physical, emotional, and spiritual feelings and behaviors. These can include…

- Withdrawing from social activities.
- Difficulty thinking and concentrating.
- Restlessness and agitation.
- Changes in eating habits.
- Sadness.
- Dreams of the deceased.
- Trouble sleeping.
- Fatigue.
- Preoccupation with death, events surrounding death, or the afterlife.
- Guilt for real or imagined mistakes made while deceased was alive.
- Loneliness.
- Anger.
- Aches and pains.
- Financial difficulties.
- Added household and family tasks.

## Your Turn: How Does Grief Affect You?

Make a list of the different ways your loved one's death affects your life, such as no longer being a caregiver, food shopping for one less person, rebudgeting household expenses, or a change in your daily routine. Categorize them as practical, emotional, or social. Choose the item you believe is the easiest to manage and list three to five strategies you can use. When you feel comfortable with your progress (or at least that you are moving forward), choose a second item, alternating categories as you work your way through the list.

## Allow Yourself to Grieve

Allow yourself to grieve? Of course, you can, someone you love just died. But, self-expectations and societal expectations might tell a different story. Yes, your sadness is acceptable in the first week, month, or even a few months. But then many people, yourself included, might think it is time to "get over it and get on with life."

If you work, you might have anywhere from a couple of days to a week or two for bereavement leave. After that, the company expects you back at work, to use vacation days, or to go without pay. Even then, many companies are only patient for so long. If you attend school, you are excused from class for a few days and then expected to return and quickly make up any work you missed.

Society tells us that grief is short term, and so we believe we should be fine. We take our 3 to 5 days and then expect to go back to normal functioning. If you aren't ready, you think it is your fault—that something is wrong with you because you can't move on. You push your sadness aside the best you can and keep moving, trying to achieve a sense of normalcy. Life keeps moving, and you need to go with it.

Permitting yourself to grieve means you accept that you aren't okay, you might not ever be okay, and that your life is forever changed. You don't need to dive into your grief, but you also don't need to pretend you are fine. Allowing yourself to grieve means you understand and accept that you are sad and that you will always carry sadness with you. You see every new experience from the perspective of someone who has experienced a devastating loss. Permitting yourself to grieve means you accept that you don't need to "get over it" but, instead, your job is to learn how to live with it. This acceptance frees you from the guilt and shame you feel for not getting over it.

## The Psychology of Grief

Grief is a bridge between your old life and your new reality. Your journey across the bridge might include pain, loneliness, fear, sadness, shock, confusion, anxiety, relief, comfort, love, and peace. You might jump between emotions, sometimes within minutes.

Many people find they feel guilty for being happy. They believe grief should be all-encompassing and that feeling happiness or joy is a betrayal of their loved ones. When they smile or laugh, they feel a pang of guilt and pain. They remind themselves that their loved ones are dead and they shouldn't be happy. Sometimes midlaugh, they will stop themselves and become somber. If this happens, you might wonder if there is something wrong with you. How can you feel happy when your loved one is gone? Does this mean your love wasn't as strong as you thought? These feelings are normal.

We believe we can feel only one emotion at a time. If we feel sad, there is no room for any other emotion. If we are happy, there can't be sadness. But it is possible to feel conflicting emotions simultaneously. We know this as mixed feelings. You probably accept it in different situations, for example:

- You are falling in love and feel happy; at the same time, you are anxious about the future.
- You are almost in an accident. You feel both relief and anxiety.
- You argue with your partner. You feel love and anger.

Having two emotions doesn't mean one cancels the other out. It is possible to experience two emotions at the same time. It is possible to be happy about one experience and sad about another—at the same time. The following steps can help:

- Accept you can feel two things at once.
- Identify and name both emotions.
- Acknowledge that you have these feelings.
- Think about the reasons for each emotion.
- Allow yourself to feel both emotions.

You don't have to choose which emotion you can have; you can have both. You can say, "I am happy to see you, and I am sad that my loved one died." Both can be true. You don't need to feel guilt over feeling joy or happiness because you can feel that and sadness from your loss.

## Your Turn: Mixed Emotions

Understanding mixed emotions is essential to moving forward after a significant death. Accepting that you can feel two emotions at once allows you to feel sad about the passing of your loved one, and at the same time, experience happiness over things that are currently happening. Pay attention to when you feel two emotions simultaneously. The next 10 times you experience conflicting feelings, name them.

## Death Can Challenge Your Beliefs About the World

Most people believe the world is just and that there is an order to the universe. But death can challenge your sense of morality, sense of justness, and your belief in a higher being. We believe in a natural order that says parents die before children and people die when they are old.

Deaths that don't fit into this mold, such as the death of a child, a murder, or a senseless accident, can make us question our belief systems. For example:

- Why did God allow this to happen?
- What if everything I believed is not true?
- What if everything is random and meaningless?
- What if there is no afterlife?
- Can I continue to believe in God after he allowed this to happen?
- What does it say about my faith if I question it so readily?

These questions are familiar to people of all faiths and beliefs. You believe prayer makes things better, but then you pray, and your loved one dies anyway, challenging your faith. When you view the death as senseless, your beliefs about right and wrong and justness and unjustness come into question.

People who aren't religious or spiritual can also face a crisis of identity after a hard-to-understand death if it doesn't fit their ideas of science, logic, rationality, and the order of the world.

For most people, these crises are temporary. As time goes on, original ways of thinking and beliefs come back into focus. As their grief heals, so does their worldview. Some people find their faith becomes stronger. And anyone who goes through a traumatic or monumental loss will learn something about themselves, the people and world around them, and their beliefs. When a loved one dies, everyone has scars.

## There Is Loss of More than Just a Person

Someone you loved died, and there is a hole in your heart. You are overwhelmed with sadness. As the days and weeks go by, you realize that this death affects your life in different ways.

*Relationships*: An intense emotional experience, such as a death, can strain existing relationships; this is particularly true when it is the death of a child. Because the grieving process is different for everyone, someone could misinterpret yours and think you aren't grieving enough or are grieving too much. You might also notice friends and family distancing themselves because they feel awkward, not knowing what to say or how to act.

*Routines*: If someone within your household or someone you cared for died, your habits change. The time you spent caring for or being with your loved one now feels empty.

*Responsibilities*: Your responsibilities can increase or decrease. When a partner dies, you need to take on the tasks he or she usually performed. If you were a caregiver, your responsibilities suddenly reduce.

*Finances*: When a partner dies, the money he or she brought into the household disappears. You might need to adjust your budget accordingly or find a way to increase your income.

Many people find their priorities and goals in life change after the death of a close family member or friend. Things you found important in the past might seem less so, and items low on your priority list could become more important to you. For example, some people pay more attention to their health or find ways to spend more time with their families.

Time could resolve many issues. However, there are proactive steps you can take to make the adjustment time easier:

*Reach out to others*: If you need help with finances or legal issues, talk with an attorney, accountant, or financial advisor. If you need help with household tasks, ask friends or relatives to help temporarily.

*Put off major decisions when possible*: The time after a death is emotionally draining. If you can put off major decisions for several months, you might be in a better position to consider your options and possible consequences.

*Talk to others*: Surround yourself with supportive people. Many people who have experienced a significant death find there are times they want to talk about their loved ones and times when they prefer silence. Create a circle of people who understand this. Look for support groups, either in person or online, where you can talk to people who know what you are going through.

# How CBT Helps

CBT strategies, especially exposure, cognitive restructuring, and writing, can help when working through grief. One study found CBT was more effective than supportive therapy. The study compared cognitive function in bereaved people against those who were not bereaved. It found that the bereaved have fewer positive beliefs about the significance of the world and their self-worth, and they had a higher level of irrational thinking.

## Using the ABC Chart

It might not seem like you have control of your thoughts after a death as thoughts of your loved one churn in your mind. But, as always, you have a choice—you can choose what to think and how to feel. As with other situations, the ABC chart is an excellent way to start.

*A—Activating event*—immediately after a significant loss, you might not have a specific activating trigger. Your mind continuously goes over what happened, such as the details of the death, or the last time you saw your loved one. As time goes on, triggers could include photos, mementos, places you visited together, or other reminders of your loved one.

*B—Belief*—I can't live without my partner. It is too difficult.

*C—Consequence*—this can be your new thought: it is difficult and painful without my partner, but in time, I will adjust.

One goal of CBT during the grieving process is to help you adapt to your new reality, including intense negative emotions, such as sadness, frustration, and pain. You can look for irrational thought patterns and change them to rational beliefs that are healthy negatives. For example:

| **Old Belief** | **Modified Belief** |
| --- | --- |
| Life is worthless. | Life is forever changed. |
| It is too difficult to think of my partner, so I avoid all talk and reminders. | It is painful to remember my partner, and whenever I think about her, I miss her. |
| Life is meaningless. | I will think of meaningful ways to honor his memory. |

## Talking to Your Thoughts

A typical problematic thought process used during the grief process is "should" and "must." We all have ideas of how someone, including ourselves, should act after a death.

"I should go back to work."

"I should stop crying."

"I must pull myself together."

The problem is that grief is unique. How someone else processes death and mourning has no bearing on how you do. And it takes time. Where you are in the grieving process is where you need to be.

It's hard to counter, "I should go back to work" because that isn't your problematic thought. To find your underlying concern, try asking questions and continuing the dialogue. For example:

"I should go back to work."

"Why?"

"Because people will judge me for not returning."

"Who?"

"My coworkers."

"What will they think?"

"I don't want them to think I am falling apart."

'Why would it matter if they thought that?"

"They would not respect me."

"What would happen if they didn't?"

"I would be self-conscious; I want everyone to respect me."

Keep going until you get down to the underlying belief. In this case, it would be that you are uncomfortable when someone doesn't like or respect you. You believe you should be perfect, and therefore, you shouldn't cry or feel overly sad, at least not at work. You think you should be strong, and to you, that means sucking it up and returning to your "normal" life. You can reword your original belief:

"I do not always have to be strong. This death is unfortunate, and sometimes I will cry. When I am ready to go back to work, I believe my coworkers will be understanding."

Ruminations, internal repetitive and intrusive negative thoughts sometimes get in the way of finding the underlying belief. Questions without answers or resolutions, such as, "Why did this happen to me?" can churn in your mind. Because you don't have an answer, the thought remains. It is okay to respond that you don't have an answer: "I don't know why this happened to me right now." By responding, you accept there is no answer and you allow yourself to stop ruminating about it.

## Imaginal Exposure

When faced with a painful situation, physically or emotionally, we often try to avoid it. Avoidance is a natural response; it protects us from a harmful situation. Instead of running headfirst into something you know will cause you pain, you retreat to a place of safety and security. But when you consistently avoid things, places, or people, it lowers your quality of life and prevents you from moving forward. After a significant person in your life dies, you see reminders everywhere. Some people surround themselves with reminders, finding comfort in having them close by. Other people avoid any reminder because of their fear of experiencing the pain of missing their loved ones.

Exposure therapy, as we discussed in Chapter 17, works to lessen the emotional reaction to a situation by slowly increasing your time facing it. The goal is to eliminate avoidance behavior. As you confront feared situations, your anxiety and fear slowly dissipate. Exposure therapy can be in-vivo, which refers to in person or in reality. For example, if you feared walking into a restaurant you frequented with your loved one, in-vivo exposure therapy would involve going to the restaurant, with assistance if needed, and confronting your fears.

Imaginal exposure involves imagining people, places, and situations that cause fear or anxiety. Using the example of the restaurant, you imagine yourself walking into the restaurant. Include details, such as what you see, smell, and touch. As with in-vivo exposure therapy, take imaginal exposure in steps. First, you might imagine sitting in the parking lot in your car; next, you might imagine walking in and standing near the entrance. Each time you create the image, take a step forward and eventually, imagine yourself sitting at a table and eating a meal.

During your imagined trips to the restaurant, your fear levels might increase initially. You might find it difficult to breathe, or you might start shaking. When you experience physical symptoms, such as a fast heartbeat, stop and employ relaxation strategies until you feel calm and can continue.

## Your Turn: Listen to Your Story

Create a story about interacting with your feared situation. For the previous example, you would write down or record the narrative of entering the restaurant, including all the details that come to mind. Stop the account at the place you feel your fear rises, and you have physical symptoms of anxiety. Each day read or listen to your narrative, focusing on relaxation strategies to calm yourself and, when ready, add to your story. As you continue, your anxiety levels should decrease. When you feel comfortable, try in-vivo therapy and physically enter the restaurant.

Imaginal therapy might not be as effective as in-vivo exposure; however, it is an excellent way to start your exposure therapy. Doing so not only prepares you for the situation, but it provides you strategies to combat feelings of anxiety.

## Getting Through Waves of Grief

> "Grief is like the ocean; it comes on ebbing and flowing waves. Sometimes, the water is calm and sometimes, it is overwhelming. All we can do is learn to swim."
> —Vicki Harrison

Grief never goes away. You never stop missing the person you lost, and you never stop feeling the hole in your heart. But somehow, you do learn to live with it and move forward in your life. Somehow, you learn to smile, laugh, and appreciate the love and beauty in your life. Eventually, you can think of your loved one with a smile, instead of feeling that deep pang through your heart.

Life goes on, and you make it through the day without too much pain. But then a wave comes along and knocks you to the ground. You might have been standing on the shoreline, watching the wave build and preparing yourself for its arrival. Or maybe the wave rose from the water without warning. Suddenly, you are sitting in the sand and all your heartbreak is back. Grief comes in waves, but as time goes on, the waves come with less intensity and further apart. In between, you have time to heal.

When that first colossal wave hits, it blindsides you. You thought you had gotten through the worst of it, and now you are devastated all over. You feel as if the loss happened yesterday. When the wave hits, be kind to yourself. Be patient. Remember and reemploy the strategies you used to get through your grief the first time. You will survive this just as you got through the original feelings of sadness.

Managing the waves of grief means understanding the intense feelings will pass. You get through them. In the beginning, waves come every day and sometimes, multiple times a day. As soon as you stand up, another wave knocks you down. Weeks or months later, you might notice that the waves are just as strong, but they aren't constant. Each time, you survive. And then the waves aren't quite as strong. They still come, and they knock you down again. At some point, you realize the waves are less frequent and less intense. They wash over you, and you allow yourself to feel the pain and grief, knowing that you will stand again.

## Your Turn: Writing a Letter

When experiencing a grief wave, write a letter to your loved one. Expressing your thoughts this way can be therapeutic and healing. Find a quiet area and accept there is no right or wrong way to write this letter. It is yours and yours alone. You can write about any topic, such as…

- Telling your loved one about the experiences you have had since their death.
- Sharing a favorite memory.
- How their death changed you.
- Something you miss.
- Something that causes you guilt or an unresolved issue.

Once you finish, you can file it away, keep it close, share it, or burn it to let the smoke carry the thoughts upward. Do what makes you feel better.

## Uncomplicated vs. Complicated Grief

Most people experience uncomplicated grief, which means that although they might experience it differently than others, there are universal emotions and behaviors, such as crying, anger, too much or too little sleep, or withdrawing from activities. These feelings and behaviors might last for days, weeks, or months. Many people experience them for a year, with a gradual lessening in intensity. Most people slowly return to their routines and live their "new normal." Most people learn to live with the absence of their loved ones.

But for some people, sorrow doesn't go away. This is called *complicated grief, abnormal grief,* or *chronic grief.* The official diagnosis is persistent complex bereavement disorder. There isn't a set time when someone goes from uncomplicated to complicated grief. However, generally once someone experiences all the firsts without their loved ones—such as first birthday, first holiday season, or first anniversary—the intensity of his or her grief lessens. For people with complicated grief, it doesn't. Their feelings remain as intense and debilitating as immediately after the death. They have difficulty resuming their lives and feel as if they are stuck in their grief. People with complicated grief have an increased risk of suicidal thoughts or attempts.

People who are more apt to develop complicated grief include…

- People who delayed their grief, possibly to help someone else process their grief.
- People who have disenfranchised grief, such as people who cannot acknowledge or express their sorrow because of embarrassment, pressure from family and friends, cultural beliefs, or religious beliefs. Examples include miscarriages, stillbirths, deaths of a same-sex partner, or deaths from suicide or overdose.
- People experiencing a tragic or unexpected death, such as murder, accident, or the loss of a child.
- People with a lack of family support.
- People with a history of mental illness.
- People who were highly dependent on the deceased.
- People who experience more than one death in a short time.

Some types of treatment include…

- Counseling and therapy
- Assessment and treatment for co-occurring conditions, such as depression or PTSD.

Some people find holistic mind-body therapies, such as yoga, meditation, biofeedback, and acupuncture, help by refocusing mental energies and reducing ruminations.

People experiencing complicated grief should seek the help of a medical professional.

Grief can leave us feeling devastated, helpless, or hopeless. When processing your feelings, it helps to examine your thoughts and restructure them to see yourself and the situation in a healthier way. Your family, friends, and colleagues might have a predetermined idea of how long mourning should last, but it is different for everyone. Grief typically lasts anywhere from a few days to a year, but for some people, it lasts longer. Allow yourself to experience and feel your sadness and accept your life is forever changed. Once the initial devastation of grief has passed, you might experience it again in waves, possibly for the rest of your life. Keep in mind these waves decrease in intensity and frequency and that you will survive. If you feel stuck in your grief or if you are unable to return to your normal activities, seek the help of a therapist or counselor.

# CHAPTER 22
# Physical Illness

"But my symptoms aren't in my head. My pain is real. My symptoms are real. It is physical, not emotional." When someone suggests CBT for a physical illness, you might think they are saying that you imagine or exaggerate your illness. But CBT is a useful part of treatment for a wide variety of health disorders. It increases coping skills and reduces symptoms of some medical conditions. Research shows it helps with chronic pain, heart disease, gastrointestinal problems, and high blood pressure. Traditional medicine is placing more emphasis than in the past on the mind-body connection and realizing that our psychological health greatly influences our physiological health. Doctors are willing to accept a combination of physiological, psychological, and social factors lead to illness more than they have in the past. Many medical professionals are adopting a holistic, or whole-body approach, to treatment which includes the mind-body connection.

## How Does CBT Help with Physical Illness?

Many people with chronic illnesses wake up each morning, not knowing if it is going to be a "good day" or "bad day." Medical advances brought about better treatments and longer lifespans, which increase the number of years spent living with health conditions. The uncertainty of dealing with a chronic disease can be psychologically taxing.

CBT works to develop psychological skills that you can use in managing your chronic illness. Goals include the following:

*Patient empowerment* encompasses patient education, where patients learn about their condition, how it affects daily life, and what they can do to improve quality of life. It also includes self-advocating, asking for help when needed, and recognizing behavior can increase or decrease symptoms, so patients take more responsibility for managing the disease.

*Empowering treatment* relates to treating the whole person, which means managing the physical symptoms as well as promoting changes in behaviors and beliefs. It is adopting a prohealth attitude, developing healthy habits, and improving treatment compliance.

*Increasing treatment interaction* encourages patients to take a more active role in their treatment, which could include asking questions, researching treatments, and being compliant. Changes in thought processes help you adopt the perspective of an advocate rather than of a victim.

People react differently to the same illness. One person might see himself as unable to contribute to society and view himself as a victim of his disease. Another could believe she can function, and with lifestyle changes, she can live a happy and productive life. Incorporating CBT into a treatment plan does not mean ignoring physical symptoms. They are still there, they often limit your life, and they often require attention and treatment. At the same time, you can change your perspective and therefore, improve your reaction to your illness.

## Living with Diabetes

Complications from diabetes occur most often because of nonadherence to diet restrictions and medications. Depression might, at least in part, contribute to noncompliance. It is up to three times higher in people with type 1 diabetes and two times higher in people with type 2 diabetes than in the general public, according to a study published in the *Journal of Medicine and Life*.

Because of this, CBT programs developed for people with diabetes have two arms—one that addresses treatment compliance and one that focuses on depressive symptoms. A clinical trial that showed significant improvement in glycemic control and depressive symptoms, published in *Diabetes Care*, had the following components:

- Meeting with a nurse educator to understand the role of treatment and to set goals for self-monitoring blood glucose.
- Two meetings with a dietician to set individualized diet and physical activity goals.
- Meeting with an adherence counselor to set self-management goals using Life-Steps, a standalone CBT intervention for medical treatment compliance, including cognitive and behavioral steps. These could include setting a daily schedule, reminders, and overcoming obstacles to treatment.
- Nine to twelve CBT sessions that included mood monitoring, thought and cognitive restructuring, problem solving, and relaxation training. Skill training included adaptations specific to diabetes care.
- Two follow-up sessions several months after the study concluded, with the option of two booster CBT sessions.

The results of this trial showed greater medication adherence as well as improvement in depressive symptoms and diabetes control.

Negative thoughts result in negative feelings, which result in unproductive behaviors. For example, let's say your blood sugar level was 200 on your last blood test, which was taken about 3 hours after eating (which is high). And let's say your response was: "I will never get this under control. It is hopeless. Why bother trying?" and you decide it isn't worth sacrificing, so you eat cookies after lunch. In this case, your negative thoughts led to unhealthy behaviors. The basic premise of CBT for diabetes is to change negative thoughts into something more productive. Instead of it being hopeless, you might think, "This blood test result is high. What steps can I take to lower my glucose levels?"

## Your Turn: Problem Solving to Eliminate Barriers to Treatment Compliance

Think about what you consider as the challenges of living with diabetes and why. Answer the following questions:

- How would I feel if this never changed?
- What changes need to occur for me to accept this situation?
- Is there one step I can take to improving the situation?
- What supports do I need to take this step?

Managing diabetes is daunting, but when you break it down and give yourself a single step to take, you feel more in control, which improves self-motivation.

Keep in mind, some aspects of living with diabetes won't ever change, such as monitoring blood sugar levels. If your challenging situation cannot change, focus on coping skills.

When living with a chronic disease, like diabetes, it is easy to feel overwhelmed because of the sheer number of negative and maladaptive thoughts. This is normal. Pay attention to your thoughts, and write them down. For example, you might think:

- "I am a failure because my blood sugar levels are always high."
- "My diabetes is beyond my control; it doesn't matter what I do."
- "I need to give up so much to control my diabetes. I won't ever get to do fun things again."
- "This is too much work; I won't follow this treatment."

Then, choose one thought to work on first. Answer the following questions:

- What is the evidence for this thought? What is the evidence against it?
- Is the thought based on emotion or facts?
- Am I ignoring other facts and basing the thought on incomplete information?
- Am I making assumptions?

After you answer the questions, formulate a new, balanced perspective. Write it down, and carry it with you. When you catch yourself falling back to the original negative thought, read the balanced one.

Stress also affects diabetes. If you have type 2, stress tends to increase blood glucose levels; for type 1, it could increase or decrease. Managing stress, therefore, is a vital part of managing diabetes. Chapter 15 provides detail on techniques you can use.

# Managing Chronic Pain

Traditional treatment for chronic pain includes drugs, rest or exercise, and surgery when appropriate. Medical interventions frequently work for acute pain; for example, when you hurt your knee, rest and ibuprofen often make the pain manageable, and in a few days, you are up and about again. For chronic pain, these treatments are often ineffective.

Chronic pain affects more than 50 million people in the United States and is the most frequent complaint made to doctors, according to the Association for Behavioral and Cognitive Thoughts. In the past, people with unexplained pain were described as lazy or faking, or doctors believed the discomfort was "in their heads" and frequently brushed aside the complaints. When addressed, doctors might recommend painkillers and psychotherapy.

The Gate Control Theory, first introduced in 1965 by Ronald Melzack and Patrick Wall, states physical and psychological variables affect pain perception. Both factors are "let into the gate" and processed by the brain as pain. Closing the gate involves introducing therapies to reduce pain, such as medication, exercise, heat/cold application, relaxation, distraction, and psychological factors like happiness.

In addition to physical signs of pain, Melzack and Wall included emotional, cognitive, and behavioral consequences. When the discomfort is acute and temporary, symptoms often do not need to be addressed or have temporary solutions. For example, you can alleviate boredom because of an injury by finding activities you can do sitting down. For chronic pain, however, you should address ongoing factors as part of chronic pain treatment.

The first step is to determine how chronic pain affects you. The following chart provides examples of the consequences of chronic pain and strategies that could help.

| Consequences | Strategies for Improvement |
|---|---|
| • Heightened emotions<br>• Depression<br>• Worry<br>• Anxiety<br>• Fear<br>• Tension<br>• Anger<br>• Helplessness<br>• Hopelessness | • Relaxation techniques such as meditation and deep breathing<br>• Mindfulness<br>• Validation of your experience<br>• Reframing emotional response, such as, "I can't handle the pain," to "I can take steps to reduce the pain"<br>• Focusing on positive emotions |
| • Cognitive impairment<br>• Focusing on the pain<br>• Boredom caused by limited mobility.<br>• Attitude and core assumption of, "I cannot handle this." | • Focusing on activities<br>• Social activities<br>• Cultivating a positive attitude, such as, "I can handle this."<br>• Problem solving<br>• Reframing perception of pain |
| • Behavioral changes<br>• Withdrawing from social and life-affirming activities<br>• Using pain as an excuse for not doing things<br>• Excessive complaining<br>• Poor health and nutrition habits | • Increasing life-affirming activities<br>• Exercising (based on medical recommendations)<br>• Following treatment plan<br>• Healthy eating<br>• Acknowledging and validating the pain<br>• Using distraction |

Pain is not "all in your head," but your brain does interpret the sensations, and those interpretations are not always the same for everyone. Some people have a higher pain tolerance than others. Some are pain sensitive. Scientists believe age, gender, fatigue, and how we experienced pain in the past influence our pain thresholds. It is possible to use behaviors and thoughts to lower pain levels; for example, we sometimes decrease the level of pain by distracting ourselves with an enjoyable activity.

Pain doesn't magically disappear with CBT. But it can help you better cope. When you change your thoughts, emotions, behaviors, and perceptions, you change how you relate to your pain and develop coping skills. CBT also encourages a problem-solving mentality. Instead of "I can't handle this," it suggests, "What can I do to improve my situation?" When you take action, any action, you feel more in control and are more focused on getting through rather than giving in to the pain.

CBT is not typically a standalone treatment for chronic pain. It is considered an adjunct therapy with other medical interventions, such as medication, physical therapy, weight loss if needed, and massage. Some people also find acupuncture helpful. You can work with your doctor to create a treatment plan that includes both the mind and body.

## Heart Disease

Heart disease is frequently the cumulative result of years of poor health habits, for example, smoking, inactive lifestyle, obesity, and not managing stress. Making positive changes, such as quitting smoking, changing your diet, and exercising regularly, requires self-motivation and commitment. These aren't temporary changes, such as resting for a week after the flu. These are lifelong, and unfortunately, many people don't reach the commitment stage until they are lying in a hospital bed after a heart attack.

Long-standing habits are the hardest to change, but adopting a healthy lifestyle improves your quality of life and can save your life. CBT improves health outcomes for people with cardiovascular disease because it targets behavior change and the underlying emotions and thoughts that contribute to unhealthy habits. The goals of CBT for heart disease might include…

- Developing relaxation techniques to reduce stress and anger, thereby lowering blood pressure and damage to the heart.
- Identifying and reduce obstacles to behavior changes.
- Accepting new strategies and behavior changes as a lifelong process.
- Implementing behavioral plans to improve treatment compliance.

Additionally, CBT strategies decrease depression. Researchers estimate between 20 and 30 percent of people with cardiovascular disease also have depression, and the reverse is true: people with depression are much more likely to have heart disease. Regardless of whether there is a direct cause and effect, improving depressive symptoms might improve motivation for making positive changes and lower the chance of dying from heart disease.

Some CBT techniques used in treatment for heart disease include the following:

*Stress management and relaxation techniques*: Stress management might begin with deep-breathing exercises, as outlined in Chapter 15. Some people disregard these as "too simple to help," but using deep breathing and progressive muscle relaxation daily could help lower stress and blood pressure.

*Thought restructuring*: This technique might directly address attitudes toward heart disease and treatment compliance. An example of an unhelpful thought might be, "I only have to take my blood pressure medicine when I don't feel good."

Strategies outlined in the section Affirmations in Chapter 9 can help you develop positive, helpful thoughts.

*Increasing activity and pleasurable activities*: One of the components of CBT when treating depression is increasing engagement in pleasurable activities, which has the added benefit of adding movement to your day. Scheduling at least one enjoyable activity each day might reduce depressive symptoms and improve quality of life.

*Problem solving*: CBT helps you find creative ways and solutions to overcome obstacles. The cognitive portion examines thoughts that could be preventing you from making positive changes, while the behavioral portion provides practical steps. Sometimes, completing these steps, even if you don't believe they help, leads to healthy thoughts. For example, buying a daily pill case might remind you to take your medication each morning; as you become compliant, you feel better, and your attitude toward medicine becomes more positive.

# Your Turn: Dissecting Procrastination

When you procrastinate, underlying beliefs might be stopping you from acting. For example, you think about joining a gym, but continue making excuses and putting it off. Digging down to your core belief helps determine the real obstacle. For example:

- People who go to the gym are in better shape than me.
- The instructors will judge me for my unhealthy lifestyle.
- I am going to be embarrassed there because I am overweight.
- I don't know how to use the equipment and will look stupid.
- Everyone is going to stare at me.
- I can't handle the embarrassment.

You can try to get rid of apparent obstacles, such as "I am busy," or "I need workout clothes," but until you get to the root, which might be "I can't handle the embarrassment," you continue to procrastinate. Think about one aspect of self-care that you avoid. Drill down in your thoughts to discover the real reason you put it off. Use the ABC chart to come up with alternative beliefs. In this case, they might be, "People who go to the gym are there to get into shape, so no one will judge me," or "The instructors are there to help, so they aren't going to judge me," or "People at the gym are focused on themselves and aren't looking at everyone else."

# Menopause

**Vasomotor** symptoms (VMS), including hot flashes and night sweats, affect about 80 percent of women during perimenopause. They are sometimes severe enough to disrupt sleep, cause sour moods, and decrease overall quality of life. The VMS symptoms typically last for between 6 and 12 months; however, some women experience them for years.

Medical interventions include hormone replacement therapy, antidepressants, or gabapentin. Some women use homeopathic medication, such as black cohosh, to relieve symptoms; however, these natural remedies have not been evaluated by the FDA for efficacy and safety.

Some studies show that CBT could be an effective treatment for vasomotor symptoms, including self-guided CBT. Strategies and techniques used include mindfulness, relaxation, stress reduction, problem-solving skills, and thought restructuring.

*Relaxation and stress relief:* When stressed, blood rushes to our skin, which is why your face might turn red when you are stressed or angry. It can also trigger hot flashes. When you feel a hot flash starting, be still, and take 10 deep breaths to lower your stress or emotional response. Regular practice of stress relief lowers your overall stress levels.

*Mindfulness:* Women who used mindfulness-based stress relief were less bothered by hot flashes, even if they didn't reduce in intensity, according to a study published in *The Journal of the North American Menopause Society*. When you practice mindfulness, you acknowledge thoughts and feelings without reacting to them. The women who used mindfulness during a hot flash reduced their "bother" of it by 22 percent.

*Thought restructuring:* Some women who get hot flashes tend to catastrophize the situation. For example, they might think:

- "I will never get back to sleep; tomorrow is going to be a terrible day."
- "I can't deal with these hot flashes. I will never get a good night's sleep again."
- "Everyone is going to notice; this is very embarrassing."
- "This hot flash means I am growing old, and my health is going to go downhill."

Giving in to negative thinking might make getting through the hot flash worse. You focus on the uncomfortableness, what others might think (mainly when the hot flash occurs at work or a public place), and how it negatively affects your future. Coming up with coping statements might help:

- "The hot flash will pass and then I can go back to sleep."
- "Hot flashes don't last forever."
- "Most people won't notice anything."

# Your Turn: Practice Mindfulness

Use a simple mindfulness exercise to help focus your attention on the moment and lessen the disruption from the hot flash. The practice involves using your senses.

*Five things*: Look around and notice five things. Don't judge them or focus too long on them; simply notice they are there. Try to find something you wouldn't usually see.

*Four things*: Pay attention to four things you can feel. It might be your phone, your keyboard, the table or desk, the fabric of your clothes, or your chair. Without judging, pay attention to how it feels, the texture, the temperature, and other details.

*Three things*: Listen for three things. Close your eyes if necessary, and listen to three sounds in your environment.

*Two things*: Use your sense of smell. Breathe in through your nose and notice two smells. These might be smells you don't usually detect.

*One thing*: Focus on one thing you can taste. If you have something to eat or drink, sample it. If not, notice the taste in your mouth.

Once done, you should feel grounded in the moment. This exercise does not require special equipment or a lot of time, and you can use it just about anywhere.

# Insomnia

Insomnia is difficulty falling or staying asleep. Many people have fatigue, low energy, difficulty concentrating, mood disturbances, and decreased productivity because of their insomnia. It is chronic if it occurs three or more nights per week and lasts for 90 days or more. There are prescription sleeping pills, some of which are only approved for short-term use, but many people prefer not to go that route or want to discontinue using them. The National Institute of Health indicates CBT is a safe and effective way to manage chronic insomnia. It uses a combination of behavioral changes, relaxation, and thought restructuring to improve sleep.

There are three behavioral changes:

*Sleep restriction or sleep consolidation*: As the name implies, this method restricts the number of hours you sleep and then slowly increases it. You start with the number of hours you spend sleeping each night. Suppose you go to bed at midnight and wake up at 7:00 A.M. for 7 hours of sleep. But with insomnia, you lay awake for a few hours before finally falling asleep. You sleep from 2:00 A.M. until 7:00 A.M., so your sleep time is 5 hours. Using sleep restriction, you hold off going to bed until 2:00 A.M. and still get up at 7:00 A.M.. In the beginning, you should feel tired, but you should also fall asleep faster or go back to sleep after waking. As your sleep improves, slowly start to go to bed earlier. If you notice your insomnia returning, begin again.

*Stimulus control*: Pay attention to your sleep habits for several nights, noticing actions that prevent you from getting a good night's sleep. For example, watching television, reading, or checking email and social media posts on your phone while in bed. Restrict your bedroom to sleeping and sex only. When you use your bed for different activities, you associate it with awake time. When you limit the use of your bed, you associate it with rest, sleep, and sex.

*Sleep hygiene*: If you are a parent of a young child, you spend time getting him or her ready to bed: a warm bath to relax, reading in bed, low lighting, and you probably limit their fluids after dinner, so they don't wake during the night. You know what to do, but then don't use the same method for you. Write a do's and don'ts list based on your circumstances. Your do's might include reading in a comfortable chair; listening to soft, calming music; and keeping the room dark and cool. Your don'ts might consist of avoiding alcohol, avoiding exercise too close to bedtime, and avoiding naps.

*Relaxation*: Mindfulness meditation, progressive muscle relaxation, and deep-breathing exercises are all ways to relax your body and your mind to help you sleep better. Review Chapters 7 and 8, and revisit the different techniques to find one that works for you. These are helpful if you lie down to sleep, and your mind starts churning and rehashing the day's problems.

*Thought restructuring*: Insomnia can trigger negative thoughts about sleep, the lack of sleep, and what happens when you don't sleep. Some of the negative thoughts you might have include the following:

- I must sleep for 8 hours every night.
- I cannot function if I do not sleep for 8 hours.
- My insomnia could cause other health problems.
- I hardly slept at all last night.
- I will always have insomnia.

Use a two-column chart to list your negative thoughts and helpful replacements. For example:

| Unhelpful Thoughts | Helpful Thoughts |
|---|---|
| I must sleep for 8 hours every night. | Not everyone needs 8 hours of sleep each night. My sleep needs might be less than eight hours. |
| I cannot function if I do not sleep for 8 hours. | I might prefer 8 hours of sleep, but core sleep is about 5.5 hours. If I wake up after that, I should be okay. |
| I must take a sleeping pill to fall asleep. | Sleeping pills have helped me in the past, but it is better to fall asleep on my own. As I practice the CBT techniques, I will more easily fall asleep. |

| Unhelpful Thoughts | Helpful Thoughts |
| --- | --- |
| I hardly slept at all last night. | I probably got more sleep than I thought. But, if I didn't, the worst that will happen is I will be tired today. |
| I will always have insomnia. | As I learn and practice the CBT strategies, my sleep will improve. |

Make a note of which techniques work best for you. Keep track of your sleep regularly, and if you see warning signs that your insomnia is returning, go back to using the strategy that worked for you.

# Gastrointestinal Disorders

Gastrointestinal disorders (GI disorders) include the following:

- Irritable bowel syndrome
- Chronic diarrhea
- Crohn's disease
- Diverticulitis
- Inflammatory bowel disease
- Ulcerative colitis

Although each disorder has specific symptoms, some common ones include abdominal pain, bloating, and diarrhea or constipation. These bring uncertainty and challenges to daily life and take an emotional toll. People with chronic GI conditions are more likely to have depression and anxiety and a lower quality of life than people without them.

Stress does not cause GI disorders. However, it can trigger episodes, worsen symptoms, and make it harder to treat. Negative thinking patterns might cause you to feel powerless and hopeless, especially when facing a chronic illness. Your behavior often reflects negative thinking, such as not caring for yourself, skipping medical appointments, and withdrawing from supportive people. CBT helps with recognizing and improving coping skills for stress.

There are six stages of CBT for GI conditions:

1. Education: Learning about stress, its relationship to GI disorders, and understanding the gut-mind connection.
2. Coping with stress: Identifying and developing strategies for dealing with stressful situations.

3. Relaxation: Learning and implementing relaxation strategies, including progressive muscle relaxation and deep breathing.

4. Identifying and changing distorted thought processes including catastrophizing: It is common for people with GI disorders to catastrophize experiencing symptoms.

5. Core beliefs: Identifying and changing underlying core beliefs that might be contributing to stress and distorted thinking patterns, such as perfectionism.

6. Problem solving: Problem solving focuses on strengthening abilities to find creative solutions, especially as they relate to triggers and stressors that aggravate symptoms.

# Your Turn: Decatastrophizing

People with digestive and GI issues tend to catastrophize experiencing symptoms. When you catastrophize, you exaggerate the importance of a problem and assume the worst possible outcome. One method for decatastrophizing is to question your thoughts. When you are worried about the result of a situation, ask yourself the following questions:

- What is your main concern?
- How likely is it this will come true? Can you think of times from past experiences to support why you think it will or will not come true?
- If it does come true, what is the worst that can happen?
- If it does come true, what is likely to happen?
- If it does come true, what is the chance you will be okay? (Use a percentage or "unlikely," "good," and "great.")

CBT is best known for improving psychologic conditions, such as depression and anxiety. But in recent years, studies found it improves numerous physical conditions, such as diabetes, chronic pain, heart disease, menopause, and gastrointestinal problems. Depression and anxiety commonly accompany these, which sometimes prevents someone from getting treatment or following the treatment plan. CBT works to lessen the severity of symptoms to improve treatment compliance and to improve quality of life. Because CBT is an interactive process, meaning that you are involved in what and how your therapy moves forward, it encourages you to work with doctors collaboratively, becoming your healthcare advocate. It also teaches you to be more responsible for your health by learning how your behaviors increase or decrease symptoms and changing behaviors as needed.

# PART 5

# Moving Forward

CBT is not a "quick fix." It is a lifelong process and a lifestyle change. It takes commitment and practice. You might experience setbacks along the way, such as times when you find yourself reverting to your old way of thinking and old habits. This is normal. In this section, we give you the tools you need to maintain your progress and pull yourself back from temporary setbacks. We help you make CBT part of your daily life.

Should you decide this book isn't enough and want to work with a therapist, we provide information on where to find online or in-person programs and therapists. We explain the different types of therapy and give you an idea of what to expect during a typical CBT therapy session. You might want to bring this book to your therapy session, so you and your therapist can work through the sections most relevant to your life. You can work together to decide which exercises are most appropriate for your situation.

# CHAPTER 23
# Knocking Down Obstacles to Progress

You spent weeks reading this book, completing the exercises, and your progress seems stalled or nonexistent. You feel worse than when you started. Before giving up, look for reasons why CBT isn't working as well as you hoped. In this chapter, you learn about some of the common reasons CBT doesn't work and steps you can take to overcome obstacles and continue moving forward.

## Uncovering More Problems and Feeling Overwhelmed

When you use CBT, you pay attention to negative thoughts, feelings, and behaviors to change them. In the beginning, it is easy to become overwhelmed. It seems as if you "opened a can of worms," and you wonder if it would be better if you weren't aware of all those negative thoughts and feelings running through your mind. Instead of feeling better, you feel worse. You now realize how often negative thoughts pop into your head. You don't like yourself as much and feel more self-conscious and hopeless.

There is a battle going on inside your mind. On one side, you continue to make a conscious effort to improve. You notice thoughts, challenge them, and create a more balanced view of the situation. On the other side, you feel powerless to change. You berate yourself for even trying. Part of you wants to keep trying, and part of you doesn't see the point.

Numerous studies show CBT is effective at treating some emotional disorders, such as depression and anxiety. It helps reduce stress and improve self-image. However, CBT takes commitment and hard work. It isn't a miracle cure and doesn't work overnight. For a short time, you could feel worse. When you first start, you might not believe or feel connected to your new thoughts. However if you keep at it, you allow your brain to adjust to a new way of thinking and acting. Continue to work through the exercises and commit to looking at your thought processes and finding ways to change your perspective. There are no easy answers; changing for the better takes dedication and hard work.

It might help to view CBT as a lifestyle change rather than a standalone therapy. You might increase the benefits of CBT by making conscious decisions to live a healthy life by…

- Exercising, eating right, and getting enough sleep.
- Connecting with other people regularly.
- Scheduling time for relaxation and enjoyable activities every day.

## Common Reasons CBT Doesn't Work

CBT is a new skill and a new way of thinking. You will make mistakes and experience setbacks. The following sections outline some of the common reasons CBT doesn't work as effectively as it could. Look through these to see if any relate to your situation.

### You Don't Practice

It took you years of negative thinking to get where you are today. You don't need years to undo these thought processes, but you do need to practice. When you challenge negative thinking, saying or reading a new thought doesn't mean you believe it. But when you repeatedly say it aloud, you begin to accept it. Think back to learning to ride a bike. You didn't climb on the bike and take off; you had to practice, fall, get up, and do it again. Some people learn quicker than others. Some need more time to keep the bike upright and ride down the street. CBT is the same. The results improve with practice and repetition.

Suppose your boss gives you a project to complete. You believe the deadline is unreasonable. Your first thought is, "I am never going to get this done on time." Your motivation plummets. When you realize your negative thinking affects your behavior, you challenge it, remembering other times you have completed projects within short time frames. You rephrase your thought to, "Getting this done in a short time could be tough, but I can do it." You repeat this thought, emphasizing the "I can do it" part. As you repeat the phrase, you increase motivation.

When you challenge your thinking and create new thoughts or perceptions, write them down. Post it on your mirror, refrigerator, or the dashboard of your car. Keep a copy with you and read it aloud throughout the day. Repetition is key.

As you work through the different techniques, don't forget to practice the skills you already learned. Set aside time each week to review them by reviewing the completed exercises and thinking about times you used the strategies in real-life situations. Congratulate yourself on your progress.

## You Believe Self-Acceptance Means Not Changing

In CBT, you practice self-acceptance. You learn to appreciate your whole self and understand you make mistakes. You accept errors and move on without allowing them to define you. Some people view this as an excuse not to change, thinking, "I made a mistake; that is okay." But there is a difference between "I made a mistake. I am human," and "I made a mistake. What can I learn from this experience, and how can I improve next time?" CBT is not an excuse for remaining stuck. When practiced and incorporated into your daily life, it helps you make healthier choices in how you think and behave.

## You Try to Eliminate Emotions

Many of the exercises in this book work by removing emotion to look at a situation objectively, so you can react based on facts instead of feelings. It doesn't mean you should try to be emotionless. As explained in Chapter 4, emotions are neither good nor bad; they merely reflect how you feel and think. It is your reaction to the feeling and situation that is positive or negative.

You can't eliminate your emotions. You need them to interpret the world around you. They raise a flag to let you know that something is amiss. CBT doesn't teach you to ignore your emotions; it teaches you to reflect on your feeling and then intellectually choose the best response.

## You Assume Learning CBT Is Enough

You have read through the book, and the concepts make sense to you. You can even name a few negative thoughts from the past day. And that, you believe, is enough. Now, your thinking will become more positive. You will focus on the problem, restructure your thoughts, and improve your life.

Learning CBT is just the first step. It is up to you to put the new skills into practice and the new concepts into action. For example, suppose you want to learn to bowl. You've never done it before, so you watch videos and read a book on how to bowl. You are ready! But when you go to the bowling alley, you completely bomb. Why? Because learning how to do something is not the same as doing it. It might take you 100 or 1,000 practice games of bowling for you to be satisfied with your score.

Indeed, it is essential to learn and understand the concepts behind CBT. But creating change in your life takes practice. Suppose you often assume you know what another person is thinking. You completed an ABCD chart and now see the errors in your thinking. You are one step closer to completing the process of changing your thought process, but you aren't there yet. It won't happen automatically until you repeatedly use CBT techniques.

As you practice the exercises, you might notice a pattern. First, you stumble through them, thinking about each answer. Then, the process gets more comfortable, and you can quickly complete an ABCD chart. Soon, you can run through the process in your mind. Finally, you might find that you move from the first to the last steps without thinking about the steps in between. It is now automatic.

Some studies show that completing homework or practicing skills has a direct correlation to both the effectiveness of CBT and how quickly it works. When deciding how much time to spend on the exercises and practicing strategies in real-life situations, consider that studies indicate the more, the better. Studies show that clients who did the most homework had the best outcomes.

There is no right or wrong length of time it takes to go through this process. Everyone is different. Keep practicing and putting the concepts into practice every day, and it becomes automatic.

## You Analyze Everything You Think

Sometimes, CBT doesn't work because you use it too much. You don't say or react to anything without first taking time to analyze your thoughts. Every decision is rational and emotionless. While it is essential to be on the lookout for negative thought processes, you don't need to analyze every thought. Imagine you are driving on a road you have never been on before. You have a passing thought of having a car accident. You quickly dismiss it and continue your trip. Although it is technically concerned with a future event, it doesn't need to be analyzed. It is a passing thought.

When you have a negative thought or emotion, stop to determine if you need to challenge it. For example, suppose you feel sad because a friend is moving out of the area. This is normal; you don't need to test it. On the other hand, if your friend cancels lunch but reschedules for next week and you become angry or depressed, you should challenge these thoughts because your emotion doesn't match the situation. Remember, not all negative emotions are wrong. You choose which thoughts and feelings to challenge. CBT is about finding the ones interfering with your ability to function or enjoy life.

## You Think Someone Else Caused Your Problems

Many people in therapy believe someone—parents, bullies, and the like—caused their problems. It seems unfair that you are in treatment, and they are not. You didn't want therapy—you want them punished. Now, you do the hard work, face upsetting issues, bear the cost, and waste your time. For some, getting better takes away the intensity of past events and minimizes them. CBT teaches you that although someone's behaviors caused you harm, it is your interpretation of the events that continue to cause unhelpful thinking. Doing the exercises helps you reframe your thoughts about the incident.

When someone else caused physical pain or emotional hurt, some people see themselves as a victim, which you could be. Being a victim has benefits—attention, being in the right, and using withholding forgiveness as power. Your anger, resentment, and indignation give you a sense of control that you don't want to give up. Some people see everyone as the perpetrator and view the world as an unsafe place. But continuing to be the victim can hold you back.

## You Expect an Instant Cure

CBT doesn't work overnight. You can't use one technique or challenge one thought and miraculously think in healthy ways. CBT takes work, commitment, repetition, and practice. The average number of CBT sessions with a therapist is 16. When using this book for self-directed CBT, it could take a shorter or longer time, depending on your commitment to completing the exercises and how often you practice. But no matter how often you use CBT techniques, changes don't happen overnight.

# Getting in Your Way

Years ago, there was a negative stigma attached to seeing a therapist or having emotional problems. People were labeled "crazy" or "loony." Today, we have a better understanding of mental illness, and going to a therapist is more accepted. The stigma has decreased, but it is still there. You might be ashamed or embarrassed that you "need help," believing it means you are defective in some way.

## Shame, Guilt, and Pride

Hiding problems frequently causes them to grow. It might seem embarrassing to ask for help, but keeping problems to yourself adds more emotional and physical issues. Having someone listen helps immensely, even if that person is not a therapist. Think about the people in your life. Is there someone you trust? Reach out and explain what you are going through.

You might feel guilty. Who are you to need help when so many people in the world have much bigger problems? Or you might believe your needs will be a burden to your family—emotionally and financially—which could stop you from seeking the help and support you need. Remember, you are important. Your wellbeing is important. Chances are there are people in your life who will assist you. Reach out and let others know how you feel.

Pride also gets in the way. You might think…

- I am emotionally healthy; self-help and therapy are for weak people.
- I can work this out on my own; I don't need anyone to help me.
- I don't go to doctors.

Pride sometimes masks shame. You believe people who need help are weak; if you need assistance, it makes you soft. You might think it is better to suffer than to ask for help. Remember, reaching out for help is a sign of strength, not weakness. Everyone needs help some time in their lives.

## The Fear of Being Uncomfortable

Wouldn't it be nice if everything in life was pleasant and no one felt pain, sadness, or fear? Unfortunately, life doesn't work that way. Uncomfortable feelings are a normal part of life. You can try, but you can't avoid them. In CBT, you face fears and other unpleasant emotions, which help you understand that emotional discomfort is okay. As you confront problems, you work through uncomfortable feelings to find solutions.

When facing possible fear or pain, you might move into "all or nothing" thinking, believing that if you are not ready to complete the entire exercise, you shouldn't try. Instead, break it into steps. Commit to doing just the first step. Commit to changing one thought or one action. Each journey begins with a single step. When you take one step, the second one is a little easier.

One way some people sabotage their progress is by avoiding exercises that might cause discomfort. This behavior reinforces negative feelings because when you avoid something, you strengthen the belief it is harmful and a threat to your well-being. However, to start feeling better, you must go through some discomfort. Accepting and learning to tolerate the uncomfortable feeling helps you manage stressful situations throughout your life.

## The Fear of Failure

Some people don't want to put effort into improving themselves. They think if they try and it doesn't work, it proves they are hopeless. For them, it is easier not to try. If this is you, you might read the information in this book but ignore the exercises. It is easier to believe it didn't work than to say you tried and failed. Hopelessness is a sign of depression. If you think there is nothing that can make you feel better, reach out to talk to someone.

# Your Turn: Find Your Motivation

Sometimes, the process of improving yourself sounds much too complicated. For example, suppose you are lonely and would like to make new friends, but you are an introvert or shy, and the prospect of talking to other people is overwhelming. You ignore the exercises that require you to speak to other people. At the same time, you are unhappy in your present life, the process of getting better sounds too draining.

Make a list of the pros and cons of using the CBT exercises in this book.

For example:

| Pros | Cons |
| --- | --- |
| CBT is effective. | It takes a lot of time. |
| I feel better when I change my thoughts to be more positive. | Sometimes, it is depressing to think about how negative I am. |
| I can do this on my schedule. | I don't always follow through with the exercises. |

Review your list to see what stands out as important. Do you notice any patterns? Did you list more pros or more cons? Do the advantages you listed motivate you to continue with CBT?

# Monitor Your Progress

Recording and monitoring progress helps you stay motivated—schedule time each week to review your progress and set a goal for the coming week.

*Write your problem:* Write a short description of the feelings and behaviors you want to change.

Rate how much this problem interferes with your life. You can use a scale of 1 to 10 or the words "very much," "somewhat," "a little," or "not at all."

*Write down your goal:* What actions do you want to take this week?

Each week, decide if you met your goal. If so, create a new one. If not, consider breaking the previous goal into steps and using the first step as this week's goal.

# Tips to Make CBT Work for You

Are you having a hard time getting started using this book? You aren't alone. It is hard to decide to change your life, even when it is a positive change. The following are some tips:

*Just do it.* You could be waiting for the right time to start. Instead, jump in and start. Often, motivation comes after action, not before.

*Believe that change is possible.* One obstacle to progress is that you believe things will always be the same.

*Keep a log.* You could use the same inaccurate thinking in different situations. Keep a record of your thoughts and the evidence against them to refer to and remind yourself of the more balanced view you discovered.

*Change "always" to "sometimes."* Changing the word "always" to "sometimes" gives you a new perspective. For example, you might say, "Bad things always happen to me." Changing it to "Bad things sometimes happen to me," gives you hope that something good might happen.

*Keep track of the exercises you find most helpful.* Use them again in different circumstances.

*Break goals into smaller pieces.* Breaking goals down makes them more manageable and allows you to focus on each step.

CBT techniques are simple and have often been called common-sense strategies. But that doesn't mean they are easy. It takes determination and inner strength to create positive change in your life. You are worth it.

Incorporating CBT in your life is overwhelming. In the beginning, you might believe it is easier to keep your old way of thinking. Stick with it. Many CBT sessions with a therapist last about 16 weeks—it takes time and practice. Skipping exercises undercuts your goal of improving your life; you can't learn and implement CBT strategies from reading a book without practicing the techniques. If you find the process difficult or painful, you might benefit from working with a therapist.

# CHAPTER 24
# Maintaining Gains

Core beliefs develop over a long time, frequently beginning in childhood. You bury them under problematic thinking patterns, and even after you address those, the core beliefs remain. For example, suppose you are overweight. You shy away from making friends or being in an intimate relationship. You blame being overweight for your social problems, and you think, "Other people don't want to be around me because I am overweight." If you dig deeper, below the issue of being overweight, you might find that you think you are "unlikeable" or "not a nice person." You rely on the overweight excuse because it is easier than facing the real belief. Ask yourself, "Is this the real issue?"

| Situation | Negative Thoughts |
|---|---|
| Saw old classmate on Instagram | I was such a nerd in high school. |
| | People always made fun of me. |
| | I didn't have friends. |
| | No one liked me. |
| Coworker canceled having lunch together | Here we go again. I am alone still. |
| | They probably decided to go with someone else. |
| | None of my coworkers like me. |

Uncovering core beliefs might require you to move outside your comfort zone to test your assumptions. For example, if you think, "I am unlikeable," it is impossible to check this thought if you continue shying away from other people and isolating yourself. Instead, accept you have this belief, and remind yourself you can deal with discomfort to test it. You need to talk to people and try to make friends so you can find out if you are unlikeable or likable.

- No one at work makes fun of me.
- Ask someone to meet for a drink after work.

There are two types of core beliefs: those that remain stable and those that change depending on your mood. For example, when experiencing stress or anxiety, you are more apt to believe negative core beliefs; when content or happy, you do not. Feelings that change with your mood are sometimes easier to tackle because the assumption is not constant.

# Prepare for Triggers: CBT as Part of a Healthy Lifestyle

A positive attitude is associated with better health, but it also works the other way. One study found eating well, exercising, not smoking, and getting enough sleep resulted in more optimism, assertiveness, and sociability.

*The form accompanying this exercise is in Appendix C.*

In CBT, it's important to monitor yourself and respond immediately when you are backsliding. One way to do this is to create behavior markers, or benchmarks, which signal that you are starting to backslide. Behavior markers are specific behaviors that signal a return to old habits. For example, if you have depression, behavior markers might include not leaving the house for 2 days, sleeping during the day, or a loss of appetite. Knowing your behavior markers helps you notice a setback immediately.

*Always celebrate accomplishments and successes.* Take time each evening to review situations when you noticed and challenged negative thoughts. Take responsibility for setbacks, but don't get caught up in mistakes and forget to pay attention to the times you used CBT successfully.

When negative thoughts and beliefs return, face them immediately. It might be that you didn't dig deep enough to find the underlying core belief and combat it, and you need to do that now. You might notice specific triggers to backsliding into negative thinking; if so, create a plan you can use when faced with the trigger. It is also helpful to schedule time each week to review your progress and set goals for the upcoming week.

# CHAPTER 25
# Preparing to Backslide

You're almost done! Just a few chapters left, and all your problems are gone! Wait a minute; it doesn't happen like that. As we explained in the last chapter, setbacks are common. CBT is a lifetime undertaking, not a quick fix. Hopefully, you learned strategies to help you notice negative thoughts and behaviors and address them quickly. The good news is that you can't ever go back to square one. You now know more than you did before you started this book, and you can't unlearn it. By the time you complete this chapter, you will understand what a relapse is, be able to notice the signs, and know what steps to take to bring yourself back to helpful and healthy ways of thinking and acting.

## The Difference Between a Lapse and a Relapse

A lapse, or setback, is a brief return to your old way of thinking and behaving. A relapse is the recurrence of a lapse. Illness, stress, or fatigue can trigger lapses and relapses.

Suppose you have a fear of dogs. Using the exercises in this book, you learned about relaxation techniques and coping statements to help you approach a dog. If you have a lapse, you might see a dog and become frightened or cross the street to avoid the dog. When you get home, you sit down and think about what caused you to avoid the dog. You aren't sleeping well and are concerned about finances. You are tired and stressed. This stress led you to simply cross the street rather than taking some deep breaths and walking toward the dog. With everything on your mind, crossing the road seemed more comfortable. You decide you will practice your exposure exercise with dogs, so the fear doesn't build up again.

Suppose you cross the street to avoid the dog, but when you get home, you think, "I knew this would be a waste of time. I am never going to get over my fear of dogs. I am right back to where I started." You see your setback as a failure and are ready to give up. This attitude leads to a relapse, where you go back to your original thinking and behavior.

To avoid relapses, accept that lapses occur. Years of responding a certain way toward adversity isn't going to disappear overnight. There are times you revert to your original thinking and behavior out of habit. It is your attitude toward the lapse that makes the difference.

# Your Turn: Preparing for a Setback

When faced with a difficult situation and you fall back to negative thinking patterns, you might think:

- This isn't doing any good.
- I am hopeless.
- CBT doesn't work.

It might not feel like it, but this is normal. You are going to have ups, downs, and in-betweens. There are going to be times you feel terrible and times you feel great. There are going to be times you are moving along smoothly and times you are standing still. The key to preventing this lapse from turning into relapse is preparation. Accept it is coming and have a plan for it.

There are a few ways you can prepare yourself for a setback.

*Track your progress.* Track your progress daily in the beginning and move to once a week as lapses occur less frequently. Some people find it helpful to graph their progress. They give each day a rating between 1 and 10 or use words such as "very good," "so-so," "not so good," and "very bad." Then they graph their progress to give them a visual of their development. You might notice that there were times you felt "very bad," but there were also times you felt "very good," which helps you see that the bad times are temporary.

*Use coping cards.* We've addressed coping cards several times. They work well to combat specific situations or negative thoughts. Use one side of an index card to write what you are doing or thinking now, with the new, healthy approach you want to take on the back. Keep coping cards with you or in places readily seen, such as your mirror, refrigerator, or desk.

*Write down what works.* Create a list of essential points you learned while using this book and the skills you found helpful. Place reminders in areas you see each day to review this information daily.

Knowing you can have a setback and planning for it helps it remain a lapse rather than a relapse. Remember, you have a choice. You can continue to think negative thoughts, or you can choose to challenge those thoughts.

# Warning Signs and Triggers

In Chapter 24, you started a thought log specifically for lapses. You kept track of your surroundings when you had a slip. Use this information to help you determine your high-risk situations. Some common reasons for a lapse are listed here:

- Negative emotional states such as depression, anxiety, or anger
- Interpersonal problems
- Social pressure
- Feeling overwhelmed with too many tasks
- Trying to please too many people

Usually, you have warning signs before a lapse. They might be thoughts, emotions, behaviors, or physical sensations. They could also happen when the situation takes you by surprise. Imagine walking down the street, and when you turn the corner, there is a dog in front of you. You don't have time to prepare or think about how to react. Your fear kicks in.

Common warning signs include the following:

Thoughts

- Anxious thoughts
- Negative thoughts about yourself or others
- Blaming others
- Becoming defensive about your behaviors
- Paranoid thoughts
- Ruminations

Emotions

- Feelings of sadness
- Irritability or frustration
- Feelings of being a failure
- Pessimism
- Nervousness

Behaviors

- Rituals
- Overeating or undereating

- Avoiding situations
- Arguing with others and using emotional language
- Not being able to let something unimportant go

Physical Sensations

- Stomachache
- Restlessness
- Fatigue

Based on previous exercises, write down your triggers and warning signs. Continue to monitor your thinking patterns by taking 10 minutes at the end of the day to review your thinking. Choose two or three situations that occurred that day and note your thinking process. Was it healthy thinking, or did it fit into one of the problematic thinking processes outlined in Chapter 2? Each time you handle a high-risk situation without falling into a relapse, you gain confidence and add to your belief that you can do this.

List some of your high-risk situations. Think about whether you should eliminate, reduce the intensity of, or cope with the situation. Then write one or two steps to help manage the problem. You can do this for each trigger or potentially problematic circumstance to help you focus on the solution rather than the problem.

# Your Turn: Create a Relapse Prevention Plan

Relapse prevention is a process. The following is an example; your plan should be specific to your situation.

*Step 1:* Review the exercises you completed. If you kept a notebook filled with your responses, go through it, paying careful attention to those similar to the present situation. Highlight ones you found most helpful. If you didn't keep a record, page through the book and highlight exercises you can review.

*Step 2:* Review the skills needed to combat your current problem. For example:

- Use an ABCD chart to analyze thought processes
- Work on problem solving
- Work on self-esteem
- Set goals implementing solutions
- Use relaxation techniques
- Practice mindfulness

Decide which strategies are most helpful for this situation and why you believe they will work. Think about how to implement each as it relates to your current issue.

*Step 3:* Complete thought logs. Reexamine your thoughts and work on coming up with more balanced ways of looking at situations.

*Step 4:* Write coping statements. Some examples include:

- Today was a bad day; tomorrow will be better.
- This will pass.
- I can use the skills I learned.
- This is a temporary setback.
- I know what to do to stop from getting worse.
- Everyone has bad days.
- Using the skills will help tomorrow be a better day.

Write five coping statements to carry with you and read them at least five times each day.

*Step 5:* List supports to use to help you from backsliding, such as…

- Calling to talk to a friend or relative.
- Finding a support group.
- Talking to a medical professional.

# Tips for Integrating CBT into Daily Life

Sometimes you work on your skills and the exercises in this book and easily change thought processes. But when faced with a problem, everything you learned goes flying out the window. You don't remember what to do or how to do it and revert to negative thinking. Remember, CBT takes patience and persistence.

Tips for practicing CBT skills:

*Treat attempts to use a skill or a new technique as an experiment.* When you experiment, there is no failure. Design them for you to learn from the results rather than being right or wrong. By changing your perception in this way, you remove the word "fail."

*Use real-life examples in your practice.* Throughout this book, there are many different examples. Read through the exercises and complete them again, using situations from your life. Think about future problems and use the activities to gain perspective on the best way to handle the situation. (Limit focusing on issues that haven't yet occurred, as this starts a cycle of worry.) Work on a few "what if" scenarios that have a high probability of occurring to help you view the situation differently.

*Keep a list of what you can do daily, weekly, and monthly to increase feelings of well-being.* Besides CBT techniques, what else can you do to improve your physical and emotional health? Focus on your life holistically rather than seeing it in small segments. Work on integrating items on your list into daily life.

*Create a list of questions to ask yourself* when you have unhelpful or negative thoughts, feelings, or behaviors, such as the following:

- Is this thought consistent with reality?
- Is this thought rigid or flexible?
- Is this thought unhelpful?
- Can I change the wording of this thought to create a more helpful way of viewing the situation?
- Is this thought catastrophizing or overgeneralizing a situation?

Use your standard problematic thinking processes to create questions. Write questions on an index card and keep them with you. When you are feeling overwhelmed, your answers can provide information on how to change the thought.

Think of CBT like learning to play a musical instrument. You practice alone until you feel comfortable with your song. Then you go out and play it for other people. CBT is like that. Use the exercises to practice at home, by yourself. As you gain confidence in your abilities to use the techniques, slowly begin integrating them into your everyday life.

A lapse is a short-term setback; relapses last longer. Stress, health concerns, not eating right, and the lack of sleep are common triggers. It helps to create a plan to combat lapses and relapses before they happen, such as steps to identify, resolve, and prevent further slips. You might include reviewing CBT skills, reexamining thought processes, and writing coping statements. Relapse prevention is a process, not a single activity.

# CHAPTER 26
# Internet-Delivered CBT (iCBT)

Internet-delivered CBT is any program that offers CBT through a computer or mobile device. You might hear it referred to as *iCBT, eCBT, online CBT,* or *computerized CBT.* There are numerous benefits, including convenience and the ability to participate according to your schedule. For people with mobility issues or who live in rural areas, it can be challenging to find someone with experience and training in CBT; some areas might not have access to any mental health providers. iCBT can help anyone with access to the internet; even people with only cell service can use apps on their phones. In this chapter, we discuss the advantages and disadvantages of using iCBT and how to find and choose programs, and we look at some of the available options.

## How Does Internet-Delivered CBT Work?

iCBT is an effective treatment for many psychological conditions, such as the following:

- Depression
- Anxiety
- Obsessive-Compulsive Disorder
- Panic Disorder
- Chronic health conditions, especially people with depression as a comorbidity

There isn't one standard type of iCBT, but the term encompasses two primary forms—guided and self-guided. Both follow the basic CBT structure and provide similar content and internet-based materials; however, one includes connecting with a mental health professional, and one does not.

Most programs use modules like chapters in a book. The beginning modules cover necessary information on CBT, such as what it is and the relationship between problematic thought processes and thoughts, feelings, and behaviors. The next group of modules should explain different techniques and strategies; for example, cognitive restructuring, problem-solving, managing stress, setting goals, meditation, and mindfulness. Depending on the program, there could be additional condition-specific information. The final modules usually cover self-monitoring and maintaining gains. Some programs require users to complete modules in a specific order; others allow you to go through them in any order.

Typically, modules contain necessary information, suggestions for integrating the concepts in your life, stories, examples, and homework. Some have interactive activities, such as multiple-choice questions via drop-down boxes or questions for you to consider before clicking to find the answer. Some include online workbooks with the ability to record ABC charts; others might have downloadable forms. The end of the module should consist of a homework assignment and suggestions for practicing the skill in your daily life. Many programs have an assessment at the end to determine how well you learned the material.

Guided iCBT adds interaction with a therapist to the program. There are numerous ways the guidance is delivered:

- Weekly phone calls from a mental health provider
- Supportive emails sent at predetermined intervals
- Texts
- Video conferences

The interactions provide encouragement and support, and they clarify information in the modules. Before signing up, you should clearly understand how often and how you connect with a mental health provider. Some programs are "support on request," which means they are unguided, but you have the option to request support at any time during the program.

Unguided programs, also called *standalone* or *self-guided programs,* provide many of the same features as guided therapy, though without the interaction and feedback from a mental health provider.

It is vital to read through and understand how the program you choose works before you spend money. You want to be sure you are spending your money wisely and receiving a benefit. Even if it is free, check what features it includes. Unguided programs have higher rates of incompletion, so finding one that best fits your lifestyle and needs improves your chances of completing it.

# The Pros and Cons

Because CBT includes self-contained modules and clearly defined goals and is structured with minimal therapist intervention, it is uniquely suited as a type of therapy that can be used remotely. Numerous studies found online CBT effective, with guided more so than self-guided, which might be because self-guided does not have a high-completion rate. The accountability of having a therapist seems to have more positive results.

Both are helpful for a variety of conditions, including physical disorders with psychological comorbidities, such as chronic pain.

## Benefits

iCBT offers several advantages over face-to-face counseling. The first is the expanded accessibility and convenience. People can log in from their living rooms if they have an internet connection. If they are using an app, they only need cell service. People in rural areas with limited access to qualified therapists can benefit from online services.

A second benefit is that it is time focused. Sometimes, it can take months to get in for an initial appointment with a mental health provider. With iCBT, the wait time is much less. Self-guided programs typically have no wait time, and provider-guided programs usually have a much shorter wait time. With some programs, you can start after you sign up, and a therapist reviews your information and contacts you, often within a few days. You might need to make video chat appointments in advance, but the wait isn't weeks, as face-to-face therapy can take. The online portion—completing modules—can be done at a time that is convenient to the user.

Typically, the cost for online programs is much less than face-to-face therapy. As of 2020, the average fee of a face-to-face appointment ranged anywhere from $60.00 to $120.00. The length of treatment is usually anywhere from 10 to 20 sessions. Using a cost in the middle of $90.00 with 15 sessions, the total cost of therapy is $1,350. iCBT programs typically range from $50 to $150. Some self-guided programs are free.

Some studies found that adherence was lower with iCBT than with face-to-face therapy, possibly because of convenience. It is easier to sit in your living room than drive across town to go to a doctor's office. Or it could be because it is more affordable. The researchers weren't sure why, but there was a significant difference in adherence.

Only people you want to know about your therapy will know. Despite the increasing number of people who attend therapy sessions, there may still be a stigma attached to seeing a mental health professional. When you access healthcare from the privacy of your home, you choose who you tell. For people who didn't previously seek treatment because of embarrassment, iCBT is an option.

## Disadvantages

One of the most significant disadvantages of iCBT is the lack of a relationship with your therapist. Some people prefer a direct connection and feel more comfortable when they have direct access to the therapist. With face-to-face counseling, you spend time together every week. Your therapist talks to you about concerns and goals and tailors your treatment to help you reach those goals. During face-to-face therapy, your therapist can easily adjust or change the content of sessions based on current concerns; however, this isn't possible with iCBT. These programs are frequently one size fits all.

Guided iCBT, especially with video check-ins, is similar, but your therapist isn't going to know you in the same way a face-to-face counselor will. For many people, this doesn't pose a problem; however, for someone who could face a crisis and wants the ability to call his or her therapist, iCBT might not be the best choice.

It is more difficult to ask questions or get clarifications during iCBT. For self-guided CBT, this might not be possible. You need to rely on the information and examples in the modules. For guided iCBT, there are ways to receive feedback or ask questions in between check-ins, but this is dependent on the specific program. For "support when needed" programs, the option is available to receive clarifications or ask questions, but there are usually additional charges.

The self-guided iCBT programs have much lower completion rates than guided and face-to-face therapy. The main reason is accountability. In guided and face-to-face therapy, you have direct communication with the therapist, and you are more likely to stick with it. One study found that less than 15 percent of people using self-guided finished the program. However, for those who did, improvements were significant and were in line with both guided and face-to-face therapies.

One advantage is the ability to access programs from wherever you are if you have internet access or cell service. But in some rural areas where therapists are hard to find, internet or cell service can be spotty, unavailable, or slow, making iCBT programs challenging to access.

# Where to Find iCBT Programs

There are hundreds of websites and apps that provide CBT services. Some have direct access to a therapist, some have limited access, and others are standalone programs meant to provide education and self-help, directed to a specific medical condition, one aspect of CBT, or general overall information. Which one is best for you depends on your current needs. No matter which type you choose, managing symptoms of a medical condition or working on self-improvement takes perseverance, determination, and courage.

When deciding which program is best for you, quality matters, especially if you are working with a therapist and spending money to do so; for these, do your homework before deciding which to use.

Start with a list of potential programs:

- Search online for "iCBT programs" or "online CBT therapy."
- Contact your health insurance company. Many insurers do not cover online therapy; however, some do if you use an approved provider. Find out if your plan does and limitations to the coverage.
- Support group recommendations. If you belong to an online or face-to-face support group, ask if anyone is currently using an online therapist and who they recommend.
- National organizations. When looking for CBT for a specific condition, contact a national advocacy group for that condition and contact them for a recommendation. Some national organizations to contact:
  - Anxiety and Depression Association of America (ADAA)
  - National Association of Mental Illness (NAMI)
  - American Psychological Association (APA)
  - International OCD Foundation (IOCDF)

Spend time reviewing the website. Look for the following information:

- Is there a list of available counselors? Are their credentials listed?
- Is there a way to contact the company? You might have questions about billing or changing therapists. How do you call, and how quickly do they respond?
- Are they affiliated with a hospital or academic institution? If so, are there limits (such as being a patient or student) on who can use the website?
- Is the company HIPAA compliant?
- Are you charged monthly or per session? What are the fees?
- What hours are therapists available? Do they offer evening and weekend therapy appointments? Is there a way to get in touch with a therapist during a crisis?

How does the program work? While most of them are straightforward, there might be differences in procedures, such as the following:

- How are you matched with a therapist?
- Can you speak with the therapists before deciding on one therapist?
- Do they have therapists who have CBT training and are board-certified in CBT?
- Do they have someone on staff to prescribe medication?
- What can you do if you aren't happy with your therapist?
- What are the methods of communication? For example, do they offer text, phone, or video chat conferencing? Are there different charges based on your preference?

- Is their payment method secure?
- Are there refund procedures if you are not happy with the service?

When reviewing websites, use common sense. A poorly designed website or one with spelling and grammar errors is a red flag. Suspiciously low rates might indicate a scam. There are many high-quality, reputable online therapy services, but there are also low-quality or fake services. Use your best judgment and research the service, including checking with the Better Business Bureau.

## Five E-Therapy Websites

E-therapy encompasses telehealth between a mental health professional and a client using electronic communication, such as email, video calls, and messaging or a combination of different methods. It is convenient, available no matter where you are, and costs much less than face-to-face counseling.

BetterHelp (betterhelp.com)

- Available via desktop, tablet, or smartphone.
- Counselor match based on your preferences, goals, and current issues.
- All counselors have a master's or doctorate degree.
- Communications include messaging, chatting, phone, and video conferencing.
- Can get counseling anonymously; communications are encrypted; and you can "shred" any message, so it no longer shows in your account.

MD LIVE ("MDLIVE") (mdlive.com)

- Available via smartphone.
- Accepts payments from insurance companies.
- Can choose therapists based on location, insurance accepted, and specialty.
- Can schedule an appointment through the website or app.
- Communication via chat, phone, video, and email.
- Counselors are certified and vetted.

Pride Counseling (pridecounseling.com)

- Specializes in working with the LGBTQ+ community.
- Available via desktop and mobile devices.
- Communication begins with a chat on their site/app, but you can request phone or video sessions.

- Can use an alias in sessions to remain anonymous.
- Counselors have a master's or doctorate degree.

Faithful Counseling (faithfulcounseling.com)

- Christian-based counseling.
- Available via desktop and mobile device.
- Matches you with a therapist based on your initial survey.
- Can work with therapist anonymously.
- All counselors have a master's or doctorate degree and are all self-identified practicing Christians.
- Communications via site or app chat.

Talkspace (talkspace.com)

- Available via desktop and mobile devices.
- All plans include text, video, and audio messaging; Premium and Ultimate programs add live sessions.
- Video sessions are available via mobile app only.
- Chats are not always in real time, but previous chats are visible when signed in.
- Guaranteed daily response five days/week.

# Five Online CBT Programs

Online CBT programs offer all the benefits of CBT at a lower cost and provided in a convenient format. Studies have shown that online CBT is as effective as face-to-face sessions, if attended.

Online Therapy (online-therapy.com).

- Web-based only; no mobile app is available.
- Guided iCBT program; all counselors are trained in CBT.
- Communication via chat and messaging; video is not available.
- Online library of resources, including CBT worksheets and yoga classes.

Moodgym (moodgym.com.au)

- Self-guided online CBT program described as an "interactive self-help book."
- Designed to help depression and anxiety symptoms.
- Based in Australia but available to users around the world.

- Five modules are available: Feelings, Thoughts, Unwarping, De-Stressing, and Relationships.
- Self-assessment questionnaire at the beginning and end of each module.

E-Couch (www.ecouch.anu.au)

- Web-based, self-guided CBT program for depression, anxiety, social anxiety, divorce, and grief.
- Provides information and has interactive questionnaires to assess mood.
- Gives feedback based on how you answered questionnaires.
- Progress is graphed based on how you answer questionnaires over time.
- Provides information, self-help toolkits, practical advice based on CBT principles, and a workbook.

Beating the Blues (beatingthebluesus.com)

- Web-based, self-guided CBT course focusing on stress, anxiety, and depression.
- Eight sessions with three or four modules in each.
- Has written, video, and audio content with worksheets.
- Homework assignments listed at the end of each session.
- Several scientific studies found the program effective.

Learn to Live (learntolive.com)

- Web-based self-guided CBT programs.
- Separate programs available for social anxiety, depression, stress/generalized anxiety/worry, insomnia, or substance abuse.
- Assessment to help determine which program is best for you.
- Eight lessons focused on the area you chose.

# Five Helpful Apps

There are many apps that provide guidance or support on different aspects of CBT. For example, some have guided relaxation or meditation, some prompt you to record negative thoughts and come up with a healthier perspective, and others guide you through CBT exercises. Apps are convenient and are usually low-cost as compared to face-to-face therapy or complete CBT programs.

Calm

- App for sleep, meditation, and relaxation.
- Includes relaxation music, videos for mindful movement and stretching, and nature scenes to aid relaxation.
- Sleep stories.

CBT Thought Diary

- Allows you to record your negative thoughts and prompts you to come up with a healthier perspective.
- Keep track of positive experiences to uplift your mood and remind you to practice gratitude.
- Use as a daily mood tracker.

Sanvello

- CBT-based app for depression, anxiety, and stress self-help through self-care, peer support, coaching, and therapy.
- Daily check-in feature and other CBT-based activities.
- Has a community feature for peer support.
- Ability to connect with a coach.
- Can schedule a live therapy session.

What's Up?

- Uses CBT and Acceptance Commitment Therapy (ACT) for coping with depression, anxiety, anger, and stress.
- A game with 100 fun questions to help you feel grounded.
- Forums to connect with others that might be feeling like you.
- Use catastrophe scale to put your problems into perspective.
- Many additional features.

Youper

- A mental health app that employs AI technology to help you talk about and change thoughts.
- You can have text conversations with an AI assistant to help analyze and change your thoughts.

- Some features are free and include basic conversations, mood tracker, journal, emotional insights, and a personality test.
- Premium features include symptom monitoring, advanced communications, CBT techniques, mindfulness, problem solving, goals, and gratitude journals.

Internet-delivered CBT, or iCBT, includes programs you can use on a desktop or mobile device in place of face-to-face therapy. Some programs target specific conditions, such as depression or anxiety; some programs teach specific techniques, such as mindfulness, and general CBT programs. Guided CBT programs include access to a therapist; self-guided ones do not. The benefits of iCBT include lower costs, access to CBT no matter where you live, and completing the program at your convenience. Some people prefer face-to-face CBT because therapists can tailor sessions to their concerns. When looking for an iCBT program, you should verify the website's information, just as you would with a face-to-face therapist. There are many programs available, and it is essential to choose one that fits your needs.

# CHAPTER 27
# Working with a Therapist

For some people, the decision to seek counseling or therapy is painful. They might find it humiliating or feel they are announcing that they are weak and unable to deal with life's problems on their own. They might resist therapy because of a stigma that still exists. But millions of people in the United States see a therapist regularly. Some hit difficult spots in their lives; others have mental illnesses such as depression or anxiety. Luckily, the stigma surrounding therapy is not as prevalent as in the past and reaching out for help is much easier today.

In the past, people saw therapy as something "crazy" people needed, but more than one-fourth of all adults in the United States have or do seek help from a therapist. Of those, 80 percent find it useful, 85 percent were satisfied with their treatment, and more than half indicated they were very or extremely satisfied. Women choose to see a therapist twice as often as men do.

In this chapter, we discuss reasons you might want to see a therapist, and we walk you through the process of finding the best one for you. Finally, we go through what to expect during the sessions.

## Should You Seek Professional Help?

The information and exercises in this book are here to help you. Working through the different sections might be what you need to get back on track. For others, seeing a therapist makes more sense.

Following are some of the reasons you might decide to see a therapist:

- Your current problem is too severe for you to work through on your own. Your symptoms have lasted 2 months or longer and are interfering with your daily functioning. You might have times when you feel better, but the symptoms keep returning.

- You previously tried self-help programs, such as this book, and there was some improvement, but you aren't satisfied with your progress.
- Your problems interfere with cognitive tasks, such as concentration and memory.
- You used the exercises in this book, but it is hard to apply the concepts to real-life situations. You agree with the principles of CBT and have completed the activities, but you can't leap from doing the exercises at home to using them in your daily life.
- You made progress by using this book but have hit a wall and can't get past where you are now. You want to continue to feel better and don't know how to do that.
- You need someone to keep you on track. You find you lose motivation when completing the exercises and believe working with a therapist can help you stay on course.
- You find it challenging to uncover core beliefs and resolve deep-seated emotions.

Many CBT therapists use a book like this as a resource and workbook for sessions. If you started using the exercises and want further clarification and assistance, bring this book with you and ask your therapist to use it as a guideline for your therapy.

# Conventional Therapy vs. CBT

There are different types of therapy, but the two most popular are psychodynamic, also called *talk therapy*, and CBT. This book and the exercises use the CBT model of therapy. When you choose a therapist, look for one who works with the type you prefer. The following provides general characteristics of each type.

## Psychodynamic Therapy

Psychodynamic therapy has been around for a long time and is often useful. You might know it as "couch therapy," as TV and films often portray it with someone lying on a couch telling the therapist about their problems. In this approach, the patient describes his or her issues, and the therapist listens and asks questions. The therapist looks for patterns and significant events in your past that contribute to current difficulties, often delving into childhood experiences to find reasons for your thoughts, feelings, and behaviors.

Psychodynamic therapy works on the premise that you are a dynamic being, and emotional formation began in early childhood and continues to influence your present life. It sees some current problems as the results of unresolved issues from your childhood. By talking about and exploring these, you accept and resolve them, thereby resolving present difficulties.

Following are some of the characteristics of psychodynamic therapy:

- Sessions are unstructured.
- The patient sets the agenda for the session by talking about what is on his or her mind.
- There are no homework assignments.
- Therapy focuses on personal history as well as the present.
- Your relationship with your therapist is considered central to therapy.
- Treatment frequently lasts six months or longer.
- You could meet more than one time a week.

Critics of psychodynamic therapy say it is time-consuming and expensive. They object to an undefined length of treatment; some people continue therapy for years. But, it does have benefits. It provides a safe environment to talk about feelings and behaviors without the fear of judgment. It gives you a supportive person to work with when sorting out problems. For many people, this is a preferred and effective treatment.

## Cognitive Behavioral Therapy

CBT focuses on specific issues and the present time. The theory behind CBT is that irrational and faulty perceptions fuel emotional difficulties. While you might discuss your past, the main goal is to work on current problems and make corrections in thought processes. Some of the characteristics of CBT include:

- Treatment duration is between 12 weeks and 6 months, with the average course of treatment 16 weeks.
- Sessions are structured or semistructured with deviation when needed.
- You receive homework assignments to work on skills between sessions.
- You and the therapist collaborate to set a plan for each session. At the beginning of therapy, the therapist takes more of an active role; in later sessions, you mostly set the agenda.
- In the beginning, sessions focus on the present. You explore past experiences to determine your patterns of thinking and behaviors that link to core beliefs and influence present issues.
- Your relationship with your therapist is considered necessary but not central to therapy. You are a partner in your treatment, a client, not a patient.
- Treatment relies on goal-oriented and problem-solving approaches.
- You practice new behaviors and work on challenging old thinking patterns.

Many studies have shown CBT is as effective as medication, if not more so, for treating depression and anxiety disorders. It is a practical approach and provides skills for dealing with difficult situations. The goal of CBT is to learn skills and techniques that you can use throughout your life. You become your therapist once sessions have ended.

Critics of CBT state this type of therapy focuses on logical thinking and tries to eliminate emotions. They also believe it ignores or minimizes the history behind issues. They think changing thoughts could temporarily help problems but doesn't resolve them.

Both psychodynamic therapy and CBT have positives and negatives. Which therapy form is best for you is a personal decision.

# Finding a Therapist

For therapy to be effective, you should trust and feel safe with your therapist. It is essential you feel comfortable discussing problems, experiences, and feelings. There are also practical matters, such as office location, costs, and scheduling availability. It frequently takes time and effort to find the right therapist. There are numerous online directories to help in your search (see Appendix B.) If you want a referral, talk to your doctor, in-person or online support groups, friends, local health department, or the hospital in your area.

## Questions to Ask Before Meeting a Therapist

Once you find several therapists in your area, call or email the office to ask for a short telephone consultation. It is reasonable to request a 10-minute discussion with the therapist without charge. Before calling, check their website for answers to basic questions, such as office hours and parking. If they don't provide this information online, ask during the phone consult.

Here is a list of the essential information you are likely to find on a website or need to ask before arranging an appointment:

- How much do you charge per session?
- Do you accept insurance?
- How long is a typical session?
- Will I have the same time slot each week, or does that vary?
- Do you charge a cancellation fee? If so, what are your rules for cancellations?
- What are your qualifications?
- What training have you received in CBT? How often do you participate in continuing education on CBT practices?
- What accreditations do you have? What certifications do you hold?

- How much experience do you have using CBT? How much experience do you have treating my problem (depression, anxiety, and so on)? How many clients have you successfully treated for this condition?
- Where is your office?
- Is there safe and adequate parking? Is it accessible by public transportation? (Ask based on your needs.)
- How soon can I get an appointment?

Some questions you might not find on the website that are important to know:

- What problems or disorders do you specialize in or have experience treating?
- How much experience and success have you had in the past working with this type of problem?
- Briefly describe how you might approach my problem.

Many therapists participate in online forums, maintain blogs, or have published articles. Do an online search and read some of these, if available, before making an appointment to get a sense of the therapist's style.

Sites such as healthgrades.com have reviews for different medical professionals. Keep in mind that there are still relatively few reviews for health providers, but if there are, it might give you additional information.

You can check with your state health licensing board to ask if there are any disciplinary actions against the therapist, what the therapist's current licensing status is, and what school they attended.

Some people have a preference for working with either a male or a female therapist. While there is no "right" or "wrong," it is vital that you are comfortable. If you prefer to work with one gender over the other, consider that when choosing your therapist.

If you locate several therapists in your area, try reaching out to three to compare answers. Be sure to measure how comfortable you feel while talking to the therapist—narrow your choice based on your conversations.

If you are looking for a telehealth therapist, find out their office location. Their license should be for the state where you live. Some states offer reciprocity where therapists can practice in more than one state, but your insurance might not pay for a therapist in a different state.

Check with local universities and research hospitals as they often offer medical services at a free or discounted cost.

## First Session Discussions

During your first session, it is common to cover the necessary information. Some topics include…

- What you should expect from your therapist.
- What the therapist expects from you.
- Your reason for coming to therapy.
- Your personal goals.
- The therapist's general recommendations for someone with your problem.
- The average length of treatment for your problem.
- Recommended books and reading materials.
- A general explanation of CBT.
- Goals for treatment.

If you currently work with other medical professionals, such as a psychiatrist, discuss whether the therapist is willing to coordinate care and forward reports to your doctor.

Remember, developing a relationship with a therapist takes time. You might not feel an instant rapport or connection; however, if you feel uncomfortable or don't believe this is the right therapist, go back to your search and start again.

## Characteristics of a Good CBT Therapist

CBT is a highly structured treatment program. Some therapists might say they use CBT but don't understand how to implement it.

A good CBT therapist…

*Spends time helping you understand CBT.* The therapist should explain what CBT is, what the techniques are, and how they are used in enough detail for you to use the strategies on your own after you leave the session. They focus on the CBT model of identifying thoughts, feelings, and behaviors and define your concerns based on the terms of CBT. They are willing to discuss your fears and concerns about therapy.

*Is realistic about how CBT can help you.* If the therapist doesn't believe CBT is the right treatment or can't help you, they should refer you to other medical professionals or make suggestions for different types of therapy and explain their reasoning.

*Collaborates on a treatment strategy with you.* Because the therapist is an expert in CBT theories and techniques, they should take the lead in creating a treatment plan with a structured and focused agenda for each session. Still, you should be an active participant in determining the course of treatment.

*Sets clear, measurable goals.* Goals should contain language that allows you to say, "I have met this goal," or "We still need to work on this." Set short-term (week-to-week) and long-term goals.

*Works to help you understand the relationship between your thoughts, emotions, and behaviors.* During therapy sessions, the therapist should ask questions about your thoughts and feelings and help you go through the process of evaluating them. They work with you to challenge thinking processes, provide specific steps for you to use, and provide you with thought logs and other handouts to assist you.

*Focuses on the present day.* Your therapist should delve into your childhood and past experiences only when it pertains to your current style of thinking and behaving.

*Monitors progress throughout your treatment.* The therapist tracks and monitors your symptoms. Each session, you should answer questions, in writing or orally, on symptoms over the past week. If you have questions at any time during your treatment, the therapist should willingly answer your questions or refer you to where to find the answers.

*Teaches.* Your therapist should teach new skills as well as spend time practicing previously learned ones. Your therapist should give homework assignments at the end of every session that allows you to practice skills outside of therapy. CBT requires homework.

CBT is not a quick-fix therapy. It involves learning new ways of looking at situations and changing thinking processes. It provides skills to use for the rest of your life. From the first session, your therapist should focus on teaching you how to become your own therapist.

# Be Prepared to Participate

CBT therapists frequently provide insight into your problems. They give you their ideas of what is causing your concerns and steps to overcome it. But, that doesn't mean you let the therapist do all the work. CBT is an interactive therapy, and for it to work, you must be an active participant. Homework is the key to successful CBT. Those who complete homework assignments have a much higher chance of changing their thoughts, behaviors, and feelings.

Weekly homework assignments have two purposes. The first is to allow you to practice skills. The second is to provide you a specific strategy to use throughout the coming week. Some homework is written, such as completing thought logs and ABCD charts. Some are behavioral, such as standing up for yourself. Your therapist tells you how to do the assignment and the rationale behind the task.

There could be times you don't feel ready to do the homework. If so, discuss your concerns, ideally before the session is over. Keep in mind that some parts of therapy can make you uncomfortable—for example, exposure therapy. But if you have strong objections to the homework, it is best to discuss them rather than ignoring the assignment.

# A Typical Therapy Session

CBT sessions are structured, and they generally follow a specific pattern. There could be times your therapist believes it is beneficial to deviate from the usual structure. For example, you are experiencing a difficult problem, and you use the session to discuss possible solutions. Generally, your sessions will follow a structured format.

You and your therapist set initial goals within the first few sessions. However, the goals might change during therapy. In each therapy session, you review problems and concerns you have, and based on this information, you or the therapist might suggest changes to the original goals.

To start each session, many therapists use a standardized questionnaire or oral questions to assess your mood and provide an objective view of your symptoms. Your answers help monitor your progress; as therapy continues, symptoms should lessen.

Additional parts of the session include the following:

*Review of your week:* Your therapist asks about how you felt during the past week, as compared to other weeks. They often focus on thoughts and feelings to check your overall mood. The therapist adjusts the focus of the session based on your mood when necessary.

*Review of the previous session:* You and your therapist discuss essential points of the prior session, and talk about how the information helped you throughout the week. If you spoke about a specific problem in the previous session, your therapist should ask about the resolution.

*Review of homework:* You review homework completed during the week and discuss any concerns or problems with it.

*Discussion of issues during the week:* Your therapist might ask if there are any problems you need help to solve, and if so, incorporate them into the session.

*Discussion of the plan:* Based on the issues or current needs, you and your therapist determine priorities.

*Problem solving:* At this point in the session, there is a discussion of the current problem and work on thought analysis and problem solving.

*New skills:* If your therapist hasn't introduced any new skills during the problem-solving portion of the session, they might add a new CBT technique for you to use during the upcoming week.

*Practice/exposure:* You and the therapist might practice a new skill together, such as role-playing or imagery exposure in session.

*Homework:* You receive a new assignment for the upcoming week.

CBT works by teaching new skills and helping you process information to aid in letting go of negative emotions or seeing situations from a new perspective.

During the session, either you or the therapist writes notes and summaries of important points. Homework usually includes reviewing the information.

At the end of the session, your therapist asks for feedback. You should share anything that bothered you, ask questions about things you didn't understand, and discuss ideas for future appointments. The therapist uses this information to customize your therapy, ensuring they address your specific needs.

Working with a therapist is helpful if you need help with motivation or applying the concepts in this book to your daily life. There are two main types of therapy: psychodynamic and CBT. Psychodynamic works to uncover the root causes of difficulties. CBT uses a more practical approach for you to use now. CBT sessions follow a specific structure that includes goals, learning new techniques, and practice. Homework is required.

# APPENDIX A
# Glossary

**ABC model** The theory that core beliefs trigger thoughts, which in turn, trigger feelings and behaviors. In the ABC model, *A* stands for "activating event," *B* stands for "beliefs about the event," and *C* stands for "consequences"—what you feel, think, and do because of your thoughts.

**activating event** A stimulus that triggers an automatic thought or belief.

**addiction** The physical or psychological dependence on a substance or activity.

**affirmation** A positive statement you purposely tell yourself to develop a more positive perception of yourself, to change negative behaviors, or to accomplish goals.

**anger** A normal human emotion that occurs when you feel stress or when someone infringes on your rights, threatens you, disappoints you, or takes advantage of you. Anger can be healthy or unhealthy.

**anorexia nervosa** An eating disorder characterized by an unhealthy effort to maintain a weight far below the normal range for age and height.

**anxiety** A perception that you do not have the resources or ability to handle the current situation.

**anxiety disorders** A term used to describe different types of disorders characterized by an exaggeration of the fear response.

**assertiveness** Expressing needs, wants, beliefs, and opinions in a direct way that is respectful to you and others.

**automatic thoughts**   Thoughts that pop into your mind without your consent and are present with or without your awareness.

**assumption**   Accepting ideas are true without proof.

**behavioral experiment**   Concrete actions to prove your new way of thinking and disprove your old way of thinking. There are three types of behavioral experiments: formal, informal, and observational.

**behavior rehearsal**   Role-playing skills learned in cognitive behavioral therapy.

**binge-eating disorder**   An eating disorder characterized by a compulsive need to eat large amounts of food in a short period of time.

**black-and-white thinking**   A problematic thinking process where you categorize outcomes of events and assume things will either turn out good or bad with no in-between.

**body image**   A term used to describe the way you perceive your body.

**bulimia nervosa**   An eating disorder characterized by a cycle of overeating and then purging (through self-induced vomiting or the use of laxatives) to alleviate feelings of guilt and shame from overeating.

**catastrophizing**   A problematic thinking process where you magnify every problem and assume every situation is going to end in disaster.

**complicated grief**   An ongoing state of mourning that interferes with other areas of your life.

**compulsions**   A term used to describe behaviors and rituals you feel you must complete to relieve anxiety brought on by obsessions.

**cognitive behavioral therapy**   A therapy approach based on changing thinking processes to change feelings and behavior.

**cognitive distortions** or **cognitive errors**   See *problematic thinking process*.

**cognitive restructuring**   Process of replacing unhelpful thoughts with helpful thoughts.

**cognitive triad**   Theory that depressive disorders are characterized by negative views of yourself, your life experiences (the world around you), and your future.

**consequences**   The events that occur as a result of a behavior.

**coping statement**   A statement that counters your struggles and gets you to focus on where you have control, who you are committed to, or how you are feeling.

**core beliefs**   The beliefs you hold strongly that indicate how you see yourself and others and how you view the world.

**cost-benefit analysis**   A tool for weighing the pros and cons of making a change.

**criticism**   Pointing out a mistake, fault, or an area to be improved.

**depression**   A medical condition characterized by a profound feeling of sadness, hopelessness, and helplessness.

**dialectical behavior therapy**   A type of cognitive behavior therapy that helps patients observe and label emotional reactions.

**distortion of reality**   The inaccurate thinking processes that cause you to react irrationally or emotionally.

**distress**   The feeling of being completely overwhelmed because you perceive a situation as too much to handle.

**eating disorders**   A group of conditions characterized by an abnormal emphasis on body weight.

**emotional reasoning**   A problematic thinking process where you base conclusions about yourself, others, and the world around you on your feelings.

**exposure therapy**   The process of gradually exposing yourself to a feared object or situation, often used when treating anxiety disorders.

**fight-or-flight response**   A physiological reaction to stress that results in an increase in heart rate, blood pressure, and glucose levels. Adrenalin levels go up, preparing you to either fight the threat or flee the situation.

**flooding**   An intense and constant exposure to an object or situation until fear and anxiety lessen.

**fortune-telling**   Problematic thinking process where you make predictions about the future, often with negative outcomes, and behave based on a reality that hasn't yet happened and might never happen.

**generalized anxiety disorder (GAD)**   An anxiety disorder characterized by excessive worry and anxiety without a specific cause.

**goals**   The endpoint you are trying to achieve. Goals should be specific, measurable, and achievable.

**graded exposure**   The gradual exposure to your fears starting with imagery exposure, moving to virtual exposure, and then in-person exposure until you can tolerate the experience.

**grief**   A deep sorrow for something or someone you lost.

**homework**   Written or behavioral work to be completed between therapy sessions to reinforce new skills.

**hypotheses**   A guess based on limited information to be used as a starting point for further investigation. In CBT, hypotheses often refers to testing a thought or feeling for accuracy.

**ignoring the positive**   A problematic thinking process where you only look at the negative aspects of a situation and discredit any positive information.

**image rescripting**   A way of changing a painful memory by providing a positive and empowering ending.

**imaginal exposure**   A type of exposure therapy that uses images only to reduce fears of a situation.

**internal dialogue**   See *self-talk*.

**internet-delivered CBT (iCBT)**   CBT programs offered via a computer or mobile device.

**irrational belief**   Unreasonable beliefs about yourself that lead to problematic thinking processes.

***in vivo* desensitization**   The gradual exposure to a feared object or situation in real life.

**keynote behavior**   A defining behavior that changes your entire perception and experience in one main action.

**labeling**   A problematic thinking process where you label your behavior or other's behavior in a negative way.

**lapse**   The brief return to your old way of thinking and behaving.

**magical thinking**   When you believe that if you do or don't something, it influences your environment or the world.

**mantra**   A sound, word, or phrase used to create a mental vibration used in meditation.

**meditation**   The act of consciously clearing your mind from the barrage of constant thoughts.

**meridian points**   The energy points in the body commonly used in acupuncture and acupressure treatments.

**metacognition**  A term meaning "being aware of your thoughts."

**mindfulness**  The act of directing your attention, thoughts, emotions, and sensations to the present moment.

**mind reading**  A problematic thinking process of guessing what other people are thinking and assuming it is true.

**MUSTerbation**  A term that refers to emotional and cognitive demands placed on yourself, others, or a group of people, which uses the terms "must," "should," "need," and "have to."

**nonverbal communication**  The process of communicating with someone through nonverbal means, such as facial expressions, touch, tone of voice, body movements, and eye contact.

**obsessions**  Intrusive and upsetting thoughts, images, or impulses that repeatedly occur in your mind.

**obsessive-compulsive disorder (OCD)**  An anxiety disorder characterized by obsessions and compulsions.

**overgeneralization**  A problematic thinking process that assumes what happened once will always happen and what didn't happen never will.

**panic disorder**  An anxiety disorder characterized by unexpected and repeated episodes of intense fear accompanied by physical sensations including rapid heartbeat, sweating, and shaking.

**passive**  Accepting another person's terms without stating your own needs or wants.

**passive-aggressive**  Agreeing with someone while feeling resentful.

**perfectionism**  A term describing self-imposed, extremely high standards and constantly working to attain these standards, even when it interferes with your ability to do the task or attend to other areas of your life.

**personalization and blame**  A problematic thinking process where you take responsibility for events that are out of your control and blame others for events in your control.

**phobias**  An anxiety disorder characterized by an intense and irrational fear of an object, situation, or place.

**post-traumatic stress disorder (PTSD)**  An anxiety disorder characterized by intense feelings of emotional stress and fear as a result of a previous trauma.

**problematic thinking pattern**  A distorted or irrational way of thinking.

**progressive muscle relations**  A relaxation exercise where you tense and relax your muscles, group by group.

**psychotherapy** or **psychodynamic therapy**  A type of therapy focused on discovering the underlying causes and previous experiences for thoughts and feelings.

**rational emotive imagery**  The process of using imagery to practice new emotional and physical habits.

**reality testing**  Mini experiments that test your thoughts and look for facts to challenge negative beliefs and predictions by taking actions to prove your original ideas wrong.

**relapse**  A term used to denote a return to your old way of thinking and behaving.

**relapse-prevention plan**  A plan to recognize high-risk situations and effectively deal with them to prevent a return to old habits.

**rituals**  The behaviors or thoughts used to help alleviate anxiety caused by obsessions.

**rumination**  The mental act of reviewing and analyzing thoughts and situations, including why you feel the way you do.

**self-acceptance**  Recognizing your weaknesses, faults, and limitations, and accepting that these do not define who you are or your self-worth. It is liking who you are, faults and all.

**self-efficacy**  The belief that you can handle a situation.

**self-esteem**  Your opinion of your overall value and self-worth.

**self-talk**  A running commentary in your mind (also known as *internal dialogue*) that reflects and interprets the world around you. It can be positive or negative.

**"should" and "must"**  A problematic thinking process where you have strong beliefs about how other people should act and become angry when they don't act in that way.

**social anxiety disorder (SAD)**  An anxiety disorder characterized by excessive and unreasonable fear of social situations.

**spontaneous imagery**  The automatic thoughts that appear as images in your mind.

**stress**  The emotional or mental strain when you are faced with demanding circumstances.

**substance abuse**  A dependence on an addictive substance, such as alcohol or drugs.

**systematic desensitization**  A gradual exposure to a feared object or situation.

**thought log**  A written record of your thoughts and feelings.

**trigger**   A stimulus that causes a thought or behavior.

**uncomplicated grief**   Refers to the normal grieving process.

**virtual exposure**   A type of exposure therapy using computer-generated images and videos.

**visualization**   The act of using your imagination to create mental pictures and images.

# APPENDIX B
# Resources for Finding a CBT Therapist

## National Organizations

**Academy of Cognitive Therapy**
245 N. 15th St., MS 403
17 New College Building
Philadelphia, PA 19102
academyofct.org

**Association for Behavioral and Cognitive Therapies**
305 7th Ave.
16th Floor
New York, NY 10001
212-647-1890
abct.org

**International Association for Cognitive Psychotherapy**
the-iacp.com

**National Association of Cognitive-Behavioral Therapists**
P.O. Box 2195
Weirton, WV 26062
800-253-0167
nacbt.org

## Resources for Specific Issues

**Anorexia Nervosa and Related Eating Disorders, Inc.**
anred.com

**Anxiety and Depression Association of America**
8701 George Ave.
Suite 412
Silver Spring, MD 20910
240-485-1001
adaa.org

**Depression and Bipolar Support Alliance**
55 E. Jackson Blvd.
Suite 490
Chicago, IL 60654
800-826-3632
dbsalliance.org

**International OCD Foundation, Inc.**
P.O. Box 961029
Boston, MA 02108
617-973-5801
iocdf.org

**National Alliance on Mental Illness**
4301 Wilson Blvd.
Suite 300
Arlington, VA 22203
703-524-7600
nami.org

**National Anxiety Foundation**
3135 Custer Dr.
Lexington, KY 40517
606-272-7166
nationalanxietyfoundation.org

**National Council for Behavioral Health**
1400 K St. NW
Washington, DC 20005
thenationalcouncil.org

**National Eating Disorder Association**
165 W. 46th St.
Suite 402
New York, NY 10036
212-575-6200
nationaleatingdisorders.org

**Depression.org**
4600 Campus Dr.
Suite 107
Newport Beach, CA 92660
Depression.org

**National Institute of Mental Illness**
1201 Prince St.
Alexandria, VA 22314
703-684-7722
nimh.nih.gov

# APPENDIX C
# Forms

Success with CBT is directly linked with the willingness to complete exercises, or homework, to help you practice and reinforce skills. Studies have found that those who go through CBT but don't complete homework take longer to make positive changes or recover, and they have a more difficult time putting strategies into practice in their daily lives. While you might feel like you are back in school or think that they are a waste of your time, these exercises help you get the most from CBT.

In this section, we provide many of the forms you need to complete the exercises. Some of the forms, such as the ABC chart, are used in more than one assignment or are used repeatedly. In those instances, it is noted at the top of the form. It might be helpful to make copies of these forms. If you prefer to use a notebook for completing exercises, use the forms in this section as a guideline.

The forms in this section follow one of the "Your Turn" exercises. There are additional exercises, suggestions, and activities in the book that do not require specific forms. These are useful to complete but do not have an associated form in this appendix.

It is helpful to keep your completed exercises to refer to later, so you have the information you need should you have a setback.

# ABC Chart

This form is an integral part of the CBT process. You use it in many exercises throughout this book. For some exercises, you only complete some of the columns; for others you use all six columns. Each exercise lists how to label each column.

| | |
|---|---|
| F | |
| E | |
| D | |
| C | |
| B | |
| A | |

## Questions to Ask Yourself
## Use with Chapter 3

Write down five questions you can ask yourself to challenge your thoughts:

1.

2.

3.

4.

5.

Examples:
- What emotion am I feeling?
- Where do I feel the emotion in my body?
- What was I thinking when this feeling started?
- What am I afraid might happen?
- Can I imagine myself coping with that outcome?
- What self-talk can I use to manage the outcome?

## Turning Assumptions Around
## Use with Chapter 3

Assumptions are usually quick thoughts and judgments you make without knowing all the facts. This worksheet follows the six steps for turning your assumptions around. It helps you base your reaction on facts. In the early stages of CBT, you might use this form for practice several times. Use a notebook to record your answers.

Follow the six steps for turning assumptions around. Think about each question and write your answer.

1. What are the facts of the situation?

2. What assumptions I am making?

3. What problematic thinking processing am I using?

4. Do I have any additional information?

5. Based on the information I have, what actions could I take that do not rely on assumptions?

6. Choosing my response from above, is this based on fact?

## Using Emotions to Discover Underlying Attitudes
## Use with Chapter 4

| Event | Emotion | Rating |
|-------|---------|--------|
|       |         |        |
|       |         |        |
|       |         |        |
|       |         |        |
|       |         |        |
|       |         |        |
|       |         |        |
|       |         |        |
|       |         |        |
|       |         |        |

## Ladder Rungs
## Use with Chapters 5, 12, and 17

**Most Difficult**

_____

_____

_____

_____

_____

_____

_____

**Easiest**

# Cost-Benefit Analysis
## Use with Chapter 5

| Pros (Benefits) of Continuing Behavior | Cons (Disadvantages) of a Behavior |
|---|---|
|  |  |

| Pros (Benefits) of Discontinuing Behavior | Cons (Disadvantages) of Discontinuing Behavior |
|---|---|
|  |  |

## Creating a Wish List
## Use with Chapter 7

| Enjoyable Activities (List as many as possible.) | Last Time I Participated in Activity | Most Interesting (Put a star next to two activities.) |
|---|---|---|
| | | |
| | | |
| | | |
| | | |
| | | |
| | | |
| | | |
| | | |

# Activity Journal
# Use with Chapter 7

| Date | Activity | Length of Time |
|------|----------|----------------|
|      |          |                |
|      |          |                |
|      |          |                |
|      |          |                |
|      |          |                |
|      |          |                |
|      |          |                |
|      |          |                |
|      |          |                |
|      |          |                |
|      |          |                |
|      |          |                |
|      |          |                |
|      |          |                |
|      |          |                |

## Recording Your Inner Dialogue
## Use with Chapter 9

| Time | Events/Thoughts | Positive, Negative, or Neutral | Emotional Rating (One-word rating) |
|------|-----------------|-------------------------------|-------------------------------------|
|      |                 |                               |                                     |
|      |                 |                               |                                     |
|      |                 |                               |                                     |
|      |                 |                               |                                     |
|      |                 |                               |                                     |
|      |                 |                               |                                     |
|      |                 |                               |                                     |
|      |                 |                               |                                     |
|      |                 |                               |                                     |

## Which Category?
## Use with Chapter 9

| Category | Problematic Thought Process | Counterthought |
|---|---|---|
|  |  |  |
|  |  |  |
|  |  |  |

## Testing Your Predictions
## Use with Chapter 10

A. Describe the situation:

B. What negative outcome do I expect?

C. What assumptions am I making?

D. What thoughts or facts dispute this thinking?

E. Which type of reality testing would work best: formal survey, informal survey, or observation?

Results:

New belief:

# Self-Assessment
## Use with Chapter 11

| Category | Words or statements I use to describe myself | Problematic thinking processes used for negative self-evaluation | Balanced or positive view | Words or statements I use to describe myself using a balanced and positive view |
|---|---|---|---|---|
| Physical appearance | | | | |
| Interpersonal skills | | | | |
| Work or School | | | | |
| Problem solving | | | | |
| Creativity | | | | |
| Sexuality | | | | |
| Personal productivity | | | | |
| How others see me | | | | |

## Sharing Preferences
## Use with Chapter 13

| A: Activating Event | B: "Should" and "Must" Statements | C: Emotion |
|---|---|---|
|  |  |  |
|  |  |  |
|  |  |  |
|  |  |  |
|  |  |  |
|  |  |  |
|  |  |  |

## Problem Solving
## Use with Chapter 15

Problem:

Possible Solutions:

| Solution 1 | |
|---|---|
| **Pros** | **Cons** |
| | |

| Solution 2 | |
|---|---|
| **Pros** | **Cons** |
| | |

# Create a Stress Worksheet
# Use with Chapter 15

Situation:

Immediate reaction:

Emotion:

Evidence to support any distressing thoughts:

Evidence to disprove my distressing thoughts:

Balanced statement:

New emotion:

# Reduce Your Ruminations
## Use with Chapter 16

| Negative Event | Coping Statement |
|---|---|
|  |  |
|  |  |
|  |  |
|  |  |
|  |  |
|  |  |

# Manage Big Problems
# Use with Chapter 17

My perception of the problem:

My ability to cope with the situation:

My problematic thought processes:

More balanced view:

More balanced attitude:

## Create an Anger Log
## Use with Chapter 18

| My Pain or Stressor | What Happened | What I Thought |
|---|---|---|
|  |  |  |
|  |  |  |
|  |  |  |
|  |  |  |
|  |  |  |
|  |  |  |

## Criticism, Complaint, or Request?
## Use with Chapter 18

| Automatic Thoughts | Request and Information Perspective |
|---|---|
|  |  |
|  |  |
|  |  |
|  |  |
|  |  |

# The Real Impact
## Use with Chapter 20

**Step 1:** Perceived flaw.

**Step 2:** How this flaw limits my life.

**Step 3:** Evidence to counter my beliefs and my coping statement.

## Plan Self-Therapy Sessions
## Use with Chapter 24

| | |
|---|---|
| **Positive events and situations** | |
| **My strategies that helped the situation** | |
| **How I resolved the problems** | |
| **My problematic thinking process** | |
| **Alternative views and perspectives** | |
| **Anticipated benchmarks and behavior problems** | |
| **Preparation** | |
| **Skill I worked on** | |
| **Skill for upcoming week** | |

# APPENDIX D
# References

Allen, David. *Getting Things Done: The Art of Stress-Free Productivity*. New York: Penguin Books, 2002.

Anderson, Stephan. *Cognitive Behavior Therapy: A Step-By-Step Guide to Understanding and Implementing CBT into Your Life*. Amazon Digital Services, 2014.

Antony, Martin M., & Peter J. Norton. *The Anti-Anxiety Workbook*. New York: Guilford Press, 2009.

Association for Behavioral and Cognitive Therapies. "What Is Cognitive Behavior Therapy (CBT)?" Accessed May 2014. abct.org/Public/?m=mPublic&fa=WhatIsCBTpublic.

Baer, Ruth, ed. *Mindfulness Based Treatment Approaches*. Salt Lake City: Academic Press, 2006.

Bailey, Eileen, & Michael G. Wetter. *What Went Right: Reframe Your Thinking for a Happier Now*. Center City: Hazelden Publishing, 2016.

Beck, Aaron T., John A. Rush, Brian F. Shaw, & Gary Emery. *Cognitive Therapy for Depression*. New York: Guilford Press, 1979.

Beck, Judith S. *Cognitive Behavior Therapy: Basics and Beyond*. New York: Guilford Press, 2011.

Beck, Judith S., & Aaron T. Beck. *Cognitive Behavior Therapy, Second Edition: Basics and Beyond*. New York: The Guilford Press, 2011.

Becker, R. G. *Cognitive Behavioral Therapy for Social Phobia*. New York: Guilford Press, 2002.

Berna, Chantal. "How a Better Understanding of Spontaneous Mental Imagery Linked to Pain Could Enhance Imagery-Based Therapy in Chronic Pain." *Journal of Experimental Psychopathology* 3 (2012): 258-273.

Borkovec, T. D., & M. G. Newman. "Cognitive-Behavioral Treatment of Generalized Anxiety Disorder." *The Clinical Psychologist* 48 (1995): 5-7.

Brabeck, V. B. *Healthy Expressions of Anger.* Austin: The Clearinghouse for Structured/Thematic Groups & Innovative Programs, 2002.

Braswell, P. C. *Cognitive Behavioral Therapy for Impulsive Children.* New York: Guilford Press, 1993.

Brewin, C. R. *Cognitive Foundations of Clinical Psychology.* Hillside: Lawrence Erlbaum Associates, 2013.

Burns, D. *Positive Psychology.* New York: Plume Publishing, 1999.

Burns, David. *When Panic Attacks.* New York: Morgan Road Books, 2006.

———. *Feeling Good: The New Mood Therapy.* New York: Harper, 2008.

Butler, Andrew C., et al. "The Empirical Status of Cognitive-Behavioral Therapy: A Review of Meta-Analysis." *Clinical Psychology Review* 26 (2005): 17-31.

Centers for Disease Control and Prevention. "How Much Physical Activity Do Adults Need?" Last modified December 1, 2011. cdc.gov/physicalactivity/everyone/guidelines/adults.html.

Chambers, Richard, et al. "The Impact of Intensive Mindfulness Training on Attention Control, Cognitive Style and Affect." *Cognitive Therapy and Research* 32 (2008): 303-322.

Connellan, Thomas. *Bringing Out the Best in Others.* Austin: Bard Press, 2003.

Consortium of Social Science Associations. "NIH Conference Highlights Importance of Social and Behavioral Influences on Health." Accessed May 2014. cossa.org/NIH/nihsocioculturalconference.html.

Cornell, L. S. *Cognitive Behavioral Therapy: A Guide to Understanding the Pros and Cons of CBT.* Amazon Digital Services, 2014.

Craske, M. G. *Cognitive-Behavioral Therapy: Theories of Psychotherapy.* Washington, D.C.: American Psychological Association, 2010.

Daniel, David, Ioana Cristea, & Stefan G. Hofman. 2018. "Why Cognitive Behavioral Therapy Is the Current Gold Standard of Psychotherapy." Front Psychiatry.

*Diagnostic and Statistical Manual of Mental Disorders, Fourth Edition.* Washington, D.C.: American Psychiatric Association, 1994.

Dobbins, Mary I., Solmaz Bauk, & Janet Albers. 2018. "Therapist-Guided, Internet-Delivered Cognitive Behavior Therapy for Anxiety." *American Family Physician,* 459-460.

Dobson, Keith. *Handbook of Cognitive-Behavioral Therapies.* New York: Guilford Press, 2009.

Dryden, Windy. *Be Your Own CBT Therapist.* London: Hodder Education, 2011.

Fairburn, C., & G. T. Wilson, eds. *Binge Eating Nature Assessment and Treatment.* New York: Guilford Press, 1993.

Farhi, D. *Breathing Book.* New York: Owl Books, 1996.

Foa, E. B. "Cognitive Behavioral Therapy of Obsessive-Compulsive Disorder." *Dialogues in Clinical Neuroscience* 12 (2010): 199-207.

Forsyth, John, & George H. Eifert. *The Mindfulness & Acceptance Workbook for Anxiety.* Oakland: New Harbinger Publications, Inc., 2007.

Freedman, R. B. "What Is CBT?" National Alliance on Mental Illness. Accessed July 2012. nami.org/Content/NavigationMenu/Inform_Yourself/About_Mental_Illness/About_Treatments_and_Supports/Cognitive_Behavioral_Therapy1.htm

Gillihan, Seth. *The CBT Deck: 101 Practices to Improve Thoughts, Be in the Moment & Take Action in Your Life.* Eau Claire, WI: PESI Publishing, 2019.

———. *Cognitive Behavioral Therapy Made Simple: 10 Strategies for Managing Anxiety, Depression, Anger, Panic, and Worry.* Antonio, TX: Althea Press, 2018.

Gratzer, David, & Khalid-Khan, Faiza. 2016. "Internet-Delivered Cognitive Behavioural Therapy in the Treatment of Psychiatric Illness." *CMAJ-JAMC,* 263-272.

Guided Versus Unguided Internet-Delivered Cognitive Behavioral Therapy for Major Depressive Disorder and Anxiety Disorders (2018). *Canadian Agency for Drugs and Technologies in Health (CADTH).*

Hardy, Claire, et al. "Self-help Cognitive Behavior Therapy for Working Women With Problematic Hot Flushes and Night Sweats (MENOS@Work): A Multicenter Randomized Controlled Trial." *Menopause* (2018): 508-519.

Hebert, S. "The Importance of Proper Breathing in Managing Chronic Pain." Michigan State University Extension. December 4, 2012. Accessed May 2013. msue.anr.msu.edu/news/the_importance_of_proper_breathing_in_managing_chronic_pain.

Holmes, Emily A. "Imagery Rescripting in Cognitive Behaviour Therapy: Images, Treatment Techniques and Outcomes." *Journal of Behavior Therapy and Experimental Psychiatry* 38 (2007): 297-305.

Johnson, Alisa, Lynae Roberts, & Gary Elkins. 2019. "Complementary and Alternative Medicine for Menopause." *Journal of Evidence-Based Integrative Medicine*, doi: 10.1177/2515690X19829380.

Kadden, R. M. *Cognitive-Behavior Therapy for Substance Dependence: Coping Skills Training.* Farmington, CT: University of Connecticut School of Medicine, 2002.

Khalsa, Singh Khala. *Kundalini Yoga, Sadhana Guidelines.* Kundalini Research Institute, 1999.

Kinsinger, Sarah W. "Cognitive-Behavioral Therapy for Patients with Irritable Bowel Syndrome: Current Insights." *Psychology Research and Behavior Management* (2017): 231-237.

Lackner, Jeffrey M., et al. "Improvement in Gastrointestinal Symptoms After Cognitive Behavior Therapy for Refractory Irritable Bowel Syndrome." *Gastroenterology* (2018), 47-57.

Leahy, Robert L. *Cognitive Therapy Techniques: A Practitioner's Guide.* New York: Guilford Press, 2003.

Lee, Lewina O., et al. "Optimism is Associated with Exceptional Longevity in 2 Epidemiologic Cohorts of Men and Women." *Proceedings of the National Academy of Sciences* (2019).

Linley, P. Alex, and Stephen Joseph, eds. *Positive Psychology in Practice.* Hoboken: John Wiley and Sons, 2004.

Make Your Menopause a Positive Experience. Accessed May 2020. menopause.org/for-women/menopauseflashes/menopause-symptoms-and-treatments/make-your-menopause-a-positive-experience.

Marlatt, G. A. "Relapse Prevention Therapy: A Cognitive-Behavioral Approach." *The National Psychologist*, September 1, 2000.

Masley, Jerry. "The Role of Exercise, Nutrition, and Sleep in the Battle Against Depression." Family Health Psychiatric & Counseling Center, PC. Accessed May 2013. fhpcc.com/PDFs/RolesAgainstDepression.pdf.

McHugh, R. Kathryn et al. "Cognitive-Behavioral Therapy for Substance Use Disorders." *Psychiatric Clinics of North America* 33 (2011): 511-525.

Mohan, Amit. "Effect of Meditation on Stress-Induced Changes in Cognitive Functions." *The Journal of Alternative and Complementary Medicine* 17 (2011): 207-212.

Molnar, Danielle. *A Mediated Model of Perfectionism, Affect and Physical Health.* St. Catharines, Ontario: Brock University, 2006.

Morgan, Carla, et al. "The Effectiveness of Unguided Internet Cognitive Behavioural Therapy for Mixed Anxiety and Depression." *Internet Interventions* (2017): 47-53.

Morin, Amy. 2019. "Does Online Therapy Work? Here's What Science Says" Inc.

Morone, N. E., et al. "Mindfulness Meditation for the Treatment of Chronic Low Back Pain in Older Adults: A Randomized Controlled Pilot Study." *Pain* 134 (2008): 310-319.

The National Association of Cognitive-Behavioral Therapists. "Cognitive-Behavioral Therapy." Accessed May 2014. nacbt.org/whatiscbt.htm.

Newman, C. F. "Understanding Client Resistance: Methods to Enhancing Motivation to Change." *Cognitive and Behavioral Practice* 1 (1994): 47-69.

Nordqvist, J. "Lifelong Exercise Significantly Improves Cognitive Functioning in Later Life." *Medical News Today*, March 13, 2013. Accessed May 2014. medicalnewstoday.com/articles/257562.php.

Nonacs, Ruta. n.d. Self-Help CBT and the Management of Perimenopausal Symptoms in Working Women. womensmentalhealth.org/posts/cbt-management-perimenopausal-symptoms/.

Norton, Sam, Joseph Chilcot, & Mary S. Hunter. "Cognitive-behavior Therapy for Menopausal Symptoms (Hot Flushes and Night Sweats): Moderators and Mediators of Treatment Effects." *Menopause* (2014): 574-578.

Pantalon, M. *Instant Influence: How to Get Anyone to Do Anything—Fast.* New York: Little, Brown and Company, 2011.

Richards, Derek, et al. 2017. "Internet-Delivered Cognitive Behaviour Therapy." *Cognitive Behavioral Therapy and Clinical Applications.* 10.5772/intechopen.71412.

Safren, Steven A., et al. "A Randomized Controlled Trial of Cognitive Behavioral Therapy for Adherence and Depression (CBT-AD) in Patients With Uncontrolled Type 2 Diabetes." *Diabetes Care* (2014): 625-633.

Samuel, Bradley, et al. 2017. "Brief CBT/MI Applications for Treating Pain." *Therapeutic Communication.*

Schneider, R. H., et al. "Stress Reduction in the Secondary Prevention of Cardiovascular Disease." *Circulation: Cardiovascular Quality and Outcomes* (2012): 750-758.

Smucker, Mervin R., et al. "Imagery Rescripting: A New Treatment for Survivors of Childhood Sexual Abuse Suffering from Post-Traumatic Stress Disorder." *Journal of Cognitive Psychotherapy* 9 (1995): 3-15.

Stahl, S. T., & R. Schulz. "Changes in Routine Health Behaviors Following Late-Life Bereavement: A Systemic Review." *Journal of Behavioral Medicine* (2014): 736-755.

Stone, D., B. Patton, and Sheila Heen. *Difficult Conversations: How to Discuss What Matters Most.* New York: Penguin Books, 2010.

Teten, J. A. *A Therapist's Guide to Brief Cognitive Behavioral Therapy.* Houston: Department of Veterans Affairs South Central MRECC, 2008.

Tuckington, D. K. "The ABCs of Cognitive-Behavioral Therapy." *Psychiatric Times,* June 20, 2006. Accessed May 2014. psychiatrictimes.com/schizophrenia/abcs-cognitive-behavioral-therapy-schizophrenia.

Tuschen-Caffier, et al. "Body Image Interventions in Cognitive-Behavioural Therapy of Binge-Eating Disorder: A Component Analysis." *Behavior Research and Therapy* (2001): 1325-1339.

Veale, D. "Cognitive-Behavioural Therapy for Body Dysmorphic Disorder." *Advances in Psychiatric Treatment* 7(2001): 125-132.

Wagner, Birgit, Andrea B. Horn, & Andreas Maercker. "Internet-Based Versus Face-to-Face Cognitive-Behavioral Intervention for Depression: A Randomized Controlled Non-Inferiority Trial." *Journal of Affective Disorders* (2014): 113-121.

Wallace, Lawrence. *Cognitive Behavioral Therapy: 7 Ways to Freedom for Anxiety, Depression and Intrusive Thoughts.* Independently Published, 2016.

Walden S., Digiusseppe, & R. L. Wessler. *A Practitioner's Guide to Rational Emotive Therapy.* New York: Oxford University, 1980.

Webb, Christian, Isabelle M. Rosso, & Scott L. Rauch. "Internet-Based Cognitive Behavioral Therapy for Depression: Current Progress & Future Directions." *Harvard Review of Psychiatry,* May (2018): 114-122.

Wilson, D. V. *Overcoming Obsessive Compulsive Disorder.* New York: Basic Books, 2008.

Zetterberg, Molly, et al. "Internet-Based Cognitive Behavioral Therapy of Perfectionism: Comparing Regular Therapist Support and Support Upon Request." *Internet Interventions* (2019), https://doi.org/10.1016/j.invent.2019.02.001.

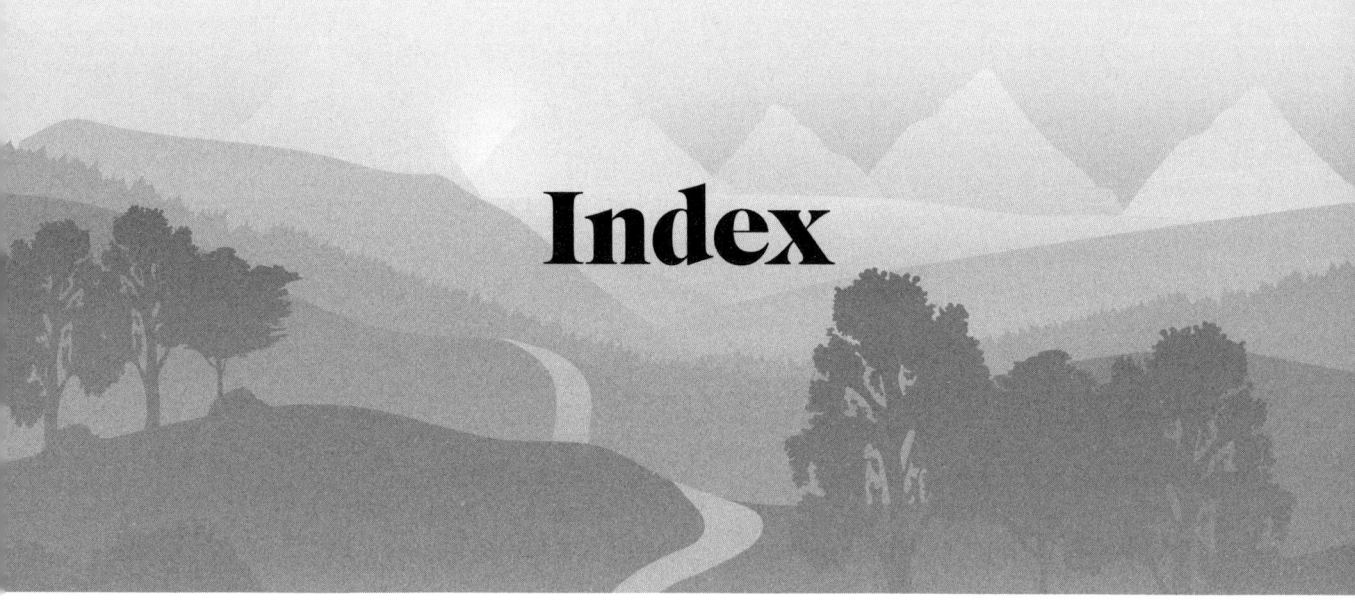

# Index

## A

ABC chart, 8–9
  additional columns, 17
  creation, 8
  grief and, 214–215
    activating event, 214
    belief, 215
    consequence, 215
  negative self-talk and, 30
  party scenario, 16
  purpose of, 8
  relationship demands, 130
  tip, 9
ABCD charts, rigid rules and, 121
ABCDEF chart, frustration tolerance, 187
absolutes, thinking in, 24
  perfectionism, 120
  relationships and, 129
acceptance and commitment therapy (ACT), 11
active listening, 33, 132
activity journal, 81
ADAA. *See* Anxiety and Depression Association of America
ADHD. *See* attention-deficit/hyperactivity disorder

affirmations, 96–98
  believable, 97
  big picture, 97–98
  lying to yourself, 96–97
  tips, 98
    counterstatements, 98
    evidence, 98
    present tense, 98
    specificity, 98
    tone, 98
aggressiveness, 135, 139
American Psychological Association (APA), 257
anger, 177–188
  acceptance of fallibility, 185–186
    example, 185
    judgments, 186
  alternate words for, 41
  anger log (exercise), 178–179
    review of, 179
    sample, 178
    scenario, 178
  causes, 179–181
    choices, 181
    counterstrategy, 179–180
    criticism or complaint, 180
    justified anger, 180
    problematic thought processes, 179–180

questions, 180
    response management, 180
complaints and requests (exercise), 181
definition of, 41
description, 177
frustration tolerance, 186–188
    documentation, 187
    exercise, 187–188
    low, characteristics of, 186–187
    low, risks associated with, 187
    problematic thought processes, 186
healthy vs. unhealthy, 181–182
    anger management, healthy, 182
    bottled-up anger, 182
    legal problems, 182
    ways of expressing anger, 182
hot buttons, 183–185
    combating, 183
    coping statements, 184
    examples, 184–185
labeling (exercise), 186
measurement of (exercise), 183
physical sensations of, 41
reframing of emotion, 185
    examples, 185
    words used, 185
understanding, 177
anorexia nervosa, 206
anxiety
    alternate words for, 41
    definition of, 40
    nervousness vs., 40–41
    physical sensations of, 41
Anxiety and Depression Association of America (ADAA), 257
anxiety disorders, 167–175
    behavior assignments, 174–175
        avoiding discomfort, 175
        uncertainty, 175
    big problems, managing (exercise), 173
        example, 173–174
        steps, 173
    common symptoms, 167

fears, facing, 169–170
    example, 169
    exercise, 171
    exposure therapy, 169
    flooding exposure, 169
    graded therapy, 169
    relaxation skills, 170
    step goal, 170–171
    systematic desensitization, 169
magical thinking, 173
physical symptoms, 167
role of CBT in treating, 168
types, 167–168
    generalized anxiety disorder, 168
    panic disorder, 168
    phobias, 168
    post-traumatic stress disorder, 168
    social anxiety disorder, 168
uncertainty, accepting, 172
    backward CBT approach, 172
    control, 172
    low tolerance for ambiguity, 172
    practice, 172
worry, problem solving of, 171–172
worry script, 173
APA. *See* American Psychological Association
apps (iCBT), 260–262
    Calm, 261
    CBT Thought Diary, 261
    Sanvello, 261
    What's Up?, 261
    Youper, 261
assertiveness, building, 135–144
    accepting criticism, 143
        first step, 143
        tips, 143
    acting assertively, 142–143
        examples, 142
        tips, 142–143
    aggressiveness, 135
    body language, 140
    defining assertiveness, 135–136
    helping others, 139
        example, 139
        frustration, 139

lack of assertiveness, 135–138
  effects on life, 138
  feelings, 138
  passivity, 138
middle ground, 138–139
  aggressiveness, 139
  being overly passive, 138
misconceptions, 144
  appearing selfish, 144
  being unlikeable, 144
  fortune-telling, 144
  nervousness, 144
  relationships, 144
rights and responsibilities, 137
steps, 136–137
  example, 136
  problematic thought processes, 137
types of assertiveness, 139
  compliments, praise, and information, 139
  conflict resolution, 141
  consequences, 141–142
  discrepancy assertiveness, 140–141
  empathy, 140
  rephrasing of assertion, 141
  self-disclosure, 140
assumptions, 31–34
  limiting, 31
  problems accompanying, 32
  tips for eliminating, 33–34
    giving benefit of the doubt, 33
    listening, 33
    past actions, 33
    questions, 33
    resisting stereotypes, 34
  turning around, 32–33
    steps, 32–33
    tip, 33
  uncovering of, 34
  unhelpful, 31
  valid, 31
attention. *See* mindfulness
attention-deficit/hyperactivity disorder (ADHD), 6
automatic thoughts, assumptions, and core beliefs, 3, 27–37, 65

assumptions, 31–32
  limiting, 31
  problems accompanying, 32
  turning around, 33
  uncovering of, 34
  unhelpful, 31
  valid, 31
assumptions, tips for eliminating, 33–34
  giving benefit of the doubt, 33
  listening, 33
  past actions, 33
  questions, 33
  resisting stereotypes, 34
assumptions, turning around, 32
  steps, 32–33
  tip, 33
core beliefs, development of, 37
core beliefs, identifying, 35–36
  analysis, 35
  coping statements, 36
  example, 35
  problematic thoughts, 35
core beliefs, rating, 36–37
first reaction, 27–28
negative automatic thoughts, 28–29
  examples, 28
  self-fulfilling, 29
questions, 31
self-talk, 28
self-talk, negative, 29–30
  ABC chart, 30
  example, 29
  incomplete information, 29
avoidance, 19
  body image, 204
  depression and, 159–160
    activities avoided, 159
    healthy behavior, 159–160
  emotional images and, 64
  grief and, 216
  perfectionism and, 124

## B

backsliding, 247–252
  CBT tips, 251–252
    experiment, 251
    holistic focus, 252
    list of items, 252
    practice, 252
    questions, 252
    real-life examples, use of, 251
  lapse vs. relapse, 247–248
    attitude, 248
    example, 247
  OCD, 196
  preparation for setback, 248
    coping cards, 248
    tips, 248
    tracking of progress, 248
    written reminders, 248
  relapse prevention plan, 250–251
    coping statements, 251
    exercises, review of, 250
    skills, review of, 250
    strategies, 251
    supports, 251
    thought logs, 251
  warning signs and triggers, 249–250
    behaviors, 249
    emotions, 249
    high-risk situations, 250
    lapse, reasons for, 249
    monitoring of thinking patterns, 250
    physical sensations, 250
    thoughts, 249
balloon breathing, 73–74
Beck, Aaron, 129, 157
behavioral experiments, 99
  creation, 99–100
  example, 100–101
  exposure therapy and, 195
  goal, 101
  OCD, 193–194
    example, 193–194
    prediction decision, 194
    repeating of, 194
  results, 100
  review of original beliefs, 101
behaviors, testing of, 101–102, 105
  example, 101–102
  expectations, 105
  feedback, 103, 105
  observation, 104–105
    example, 105
    proof of original theory, 105
  report card, 102–103
  reward, 105
  surveys, formal, 103–104
  surveys, informal, 104
benefits of CBT, 10, 266
  adaptability, 10
  length of therapy, 10
  lesson learned, 10
  measurement of progress, 10
  structure, 10
  targeted skills, 10
binge-eating disorder, 207
biological depression, 41
black-and-white thinking, 21–22, 47, 174
  body image, 201
  perfectionism, 119
blame, 18, 22–23
body image, 199–207
  behaviors, 204–205
    avoidance, 204
    body checking, 205
    external signals, misinterpreting, 205
  changing the image (exercise), 202
  definition of, 199
  eating disorders, 206–207
    anorexia nervosa, 206
    binge-eating disorder, 207
    bulimia nervosa, 206
    description, 206
  effect on life, 202
    acceptance of imperfections, 203
    scenarios, 202–203
  effect on life (exercise), 203–204
    coping statements, 204
    counter evidence, 204
    example, 203

limitations, 203
   listed of admired people, 204
exposure strategies, 204
healthy vs. unhealthy, 199–200
problem (exercise), 200–201
   statements, 200
   written list, 201
problematic thinking processes, 201
   black-and-white thinking, 201
   fortune-telling, 201
   ignoring the positive, 201
   magnification, 201
   mind reading, 201
   overgeneralizing, 201
   personalization and blame, 201
whole person, 205–206
   pie chart, 206
   review categories, 205–206
body language, 140
   relationships and, 133–134
      eye contact, 133
      mixed message, 133
      touching and smiling, 133
breathing
   balloon breathing, 73–74
   during fight-or-flight response, 72
   during sleep, 72
   mindfulness (exercise), 84
   reverse breathing, 71
   testing, 72
breathing (relaxation), 71–72
   exercise, 72
   importance of, 72
   incorrect, 71
      collapsed breathing, 72
      reverse breathing, 71
      shallow breathing, 72
   proper, 71
bulimia nervosa, 206

# C

catastrophizing, 20, 47, 137, 174
   perfectionism, 119
CBT. *See* cognitive behavioral therapy
CBT Readiness Quiz, 13
childhood experiences
   issues explored in psychodynamic therapy, 264
   myth about, 6
chronic pain, 224–226
   adjunct therapy, 226
   brain interpretations, 225
   CBT treatment of, 225
   chart, 224
   coping factors, 224
   Gate Control Theory, 224
   statistics, 224
   therapies, 224
cognitive behavioral therapy (CBT), 3. *See also* internet-delivered CBT; understanding CBT
   benefits of, 10, 266
   conditions helped by, 6
   conditions treated by, 10
   disadvantages of, 10–11
   effectiveness of, 6
   theory behind, 7–8
   therapist, 265–266
cognitive reactions (emotions), 47
   black-and-white thinking, 47
   catastrophizing, 47
   fortune-telling, 47
   ignoring the positive, 47
   mind reading, 47
   overgeneralization, 47
   personalization, 47
cognitive triad, 157
collapsed breathing, 72
common-sense strategies, 242
complicated grief
   official diagnosis, 218
   people apt to develop, 219
   uncomplicated grief vs., 218–219
compliments, 139
computerized CBT. *See* internet-delivered CBT

conditioning, 49
conflict resolution, 141
contempt
    alternate words for, 43
    definition of, 42
    physical sensations of, 43
coping cards, 61, 248
coping statements, 36
    goal setting and, 57
    relapse prevention, 251
core beliefs, 4–5
    beginnings of, 6
    development of, 37, 243
    perspectives, 5
    rating, 36–37
    scenarios, 4
    true, 244
    types of, 244
    uncovering of, 244
core beliefs, identifying, 35–36
    analysis, 35
    coping statements, 36
    example, 35
    problematic thoughts, 35
cost-benefit analysis, 123–124
    definition of, 58
    in goal setting, 59
"couch therapy," 264
COVID-19 pandemic, 191
criticism, accepting, 143
    first step, 143
    tips, 143

# D

depression, 155–165
    alternate words for, 42
    avoidance, 159–160
        activities avoided, 159
        exercise, 160
        healthy behavior, switch to, 159–160
    CBT treatment of, 156–157
        ABC chart, 157
        benefits, 156
        cognitive triad, 157
        example thoughts, 157
        medication and, 156
    "do nothing" syndrome, 158–159
        daily activity schedule, 158–159
        goal, 158
    lack of motivation, 158–159
        daily activity schedule, 158–159
        goal, 158
    major, 42
    physical sensations of, 42
    reactionary vs. biological, 41
    ruminations, 160–161
        activities to stop process, 161
        conscious decision, 161
        documentation, 161
        "go-to" activity, 161
        thoughts surrounding, 160–161
    ruminations (exercise), 161–163
        coping statements, 161, 163
        list, 162
        negative thoughts, challenge to, 162
        new thoughts, 162–163
    sadness vs., 41–42, 155–156, 165
    self-care, 163–165
        diet, 163–164
        exercise, 164
        sleep, 164–165
    statistics, 156
    symptoms, 156
desensitization, 64
diabetes, 222–223
    CBT premise, 223
    clinical trial, 222
    complications, 222
    example, 223
    exercise, 223–224
*Diabetes Care*, 222
discrepancy assertiveness, 140–141

disgust
    alternate words for, 43
    definition of, 42
    physical sensations of, 43

# E

eating disorders, 206–207
    anorexia nervosa, 206
    binge-eating disorder, 207
    bulimia nervosa, 206
    description, 206
eCBT. *See* internet-delivered CBT
effectiveness of CBT, 6
embarrassment
    alternate words for, 42
    definition of, 42
    physical sensations of, 42
emotional images, 64–65
    avoidance and, 64
    desensitization and, 64
    example, 64
    levels, 64–65
emotional reasoning, 24
emotion log, 56
emotions, 39–51
    anger and rage, 41
    behavioral reactions to, 49
        examples, 49
        positive actions, 49
    cognitive reactions, 47
        black-and-white thinking, 47
        catastrophizing, 47
        fortune-telling, 47
        ignoring the positive, 47
        mind reading, 47
        overgeneralization, 47
        personalization, 47
    disgust vs. contempt, 42–43
    embarrassment vs. guilt and shame, 42
    emotion contract, 46
    envy vs. jealousy, 43
    grief and, 212

healthy emotions
    disgust, 42
    embarrassment, 42
    envy, 43
    frustration, 41
    irritation, 41
    nervousness, 40
    sadness, 41
    stress, 43
helpful vs. unhelpful, 40
irritation and frustration, 41
learned emotions, 49–51
    conditioned emotional response, 51
    conditioning and, 49
    emotion chart, 50
    exposure techniques, 51
    fears, 50
    questions, 50
    similar situations, 51
management of, 40, 51
meta-emotions, 46
mixed emotions, 45
    example, 45
    grief and, 212
    thoughts, 45
    unhealthy reactions, 45
myth about, 6
naming, 39
nervousness vs. anxiety, 40–41
physical reactions to, 48
    complex emotions, 48
    scenarios, 48
process, 47
reframing of (anger), 185
responsibility for, 128
sadness vs. depression, 41–42
separating thoughts from, 18–19
    avoidance, 19
    blame, 18
    creating new thought, 18
    decision-making, 19
    example, 18
    negative thinking, 19
    working backward, 18

stress vs. shock, 43
thoughts and, 16
trying to eliminate, 237
underlying attitudes (exercise), 44–45
    categories of emotions, 44
    rating emotions, 44–45
    results, 44
unfairness, emotions based on sense of, 41
unhealthy emotions
    anger, 41
    anxiety, 40
    contempt, 42
    feeling overwhelmed, 43
    guilt, 42
    jealousy, 43
    major depression, 42
    panic, 40
    rage, 41
    reactionary depression, 41
    shame, 42
    shock, 43
as warning signs, 249
empathy, 140
endorphins, 151
envy
    alternate words for, 43
    definition of, 43
    physical sensations of, 43
e-therapy websites, 258–259
    BetterHelp, 258
    Faithful Counseling, 259
    MDLIVE, 258
    Pride Counseling, 258
    Talkspace, 259
exercise, reducing stress through, 151
    beginning, 151
    endorphins, 151
    as form of mindfulness meditation, 151
    recommendations, 151
exercises
    ABC chart, 18
    anger (anger log), 178–179
        review of, 179
        sample, 178
        scenario, 178

anger (complaints and requests), 181
anger (frustration tolerance), 187–188
anger (labeling), 186
anger (measurement of), 183
automatic thoughts, 31
body image (changing the image), 202
body image (effect on life), 203–204
    coping statements, 204
    counter evidence, 204
    example, 203
    limitations, 203
    list of admired people, 204
body image (problem), 200–201
    statements, 200
    written list, 201
breathing (testing), 72
depression (avoidance), 160
depression (ruminations), 161–163
    coping statements, 161, 163
    list, 162
    negative thoughts, challenge to, 162
    new thoughts, 162–163
diabetes (problem solving), 223–224
discovering underlying attitudes, 44
emotional images, 64–65
exposure, 171
gains, maintaining (behavior markers), 244
    definition, 244
gastrointestinal disorders (decatastrophizing), 232
goal setting (coping flash cards), 61
goal setting (cost-benefit analysis), 60–61
goal setting (ladder rungs), 57–58
inner narration (assessment), 95–96
inner narration (self-talk), 92–93
    cynical, 93
    example, 92
managing big problems, 173–174
menopause (mindfulness), 229
mindfulness (breathing), 84
mindfulness (diary), 90
mindfulness (practice), 86
mindfulness (thoughts), 88
obstacles to progress (finding your motivation), 241

patterns, 241
pros and cons, 241
OCD (thought exposure), 192
documentation, 192
triggering of new obsessions, 192
OCD (triggers), 191–192
during pandemic, 191
example, 191
ladder technique, 192
log, 191
perfectionism (assessment), 118–119
perfectionism (overcoming), 125
perfectionism (shades of grey), 123
physical illness (procrastination), 227
relationships, improving (sharing preferences), 130–131
relaxation techniques (activity journal), 81
relaxation techniques (breathing), 72
balloon breathing, 73–74
deep breathing, 73
feeling the difference, 73
muscle development, 73
sighing, 74
relaxation techniques (hobbies), 79
relaxation techniques (Kirtan Kriya meditation), 76
mantra, 76
meridian points, 76
relaxation techniques (meditation), 75–76
relaxation techniques (progressive muscle relaxation), 77–78
review of, 250
self-esteem (mini action plan), 114
self-esteem (self-assessment), 112
statements, 112
words, negative and positive, 112
self-talk, 28
stress, everyday (problem solving), 148
stress, everyday (worksheet), 150–151
testing predictions, 106
turning assumptions around, 32
visualization and imagery (imagery creation), 68
athletes, 68
practice, 68
visualization and imagery (keynote behavior visualizations), 69–70
worry script, 173
experiments (behavioral), 99
creation, 99–100
example, 100–101
exposure therapy and, 195
goal, 101
OCD, 193–194
example, 193–194
prediction decision, 194
repeating of, 194
results, 100
review of original beliefs, 101
exposure strategies, body image, 204
exposure therapy, 216
facing fears with, 169
goal of, 216
OCD, 194–195
anxiety level, 195
imagery, 195
list of actions, 194
ranking of situations, 195
urge to perform rituals, 195
types, 169
worry script, 173

# F

Facebook groups, 80
fears, conditioning and, 50
fears, facing, 169–170
example, 169
exercise, 171
exposure therapy, 169
flooding exposure, 169
graded therapy, 169
relaxation skills, 170
step goal, 170–171
systematic desensitization, 169
feedback behavioral experiment, 103
"feel-good" brain chemical, 151

feeling overwhelmed
    alternate words, 43
    definition of, 43
    obstacles to progress and, 235–236
        battle, 235
        effectiveness of CBT, 235
        lifestyle change, 236
    physical sensations of, 43
feelings, interpretation of. *See* thoughts and feelings, interpretation of
fight-or-flight response, 40, 43
    activation, 72
    breathing during, 72
fitness program, 81–82
    action plan, 82
    goals, 81
    research results, 81
    structured time, 81
flooding exposure, facing fears with, 169
fortune-telling, 21, 47, 137, 144
frustration
    alternate words for, 41
    definition of, 41
    healthiness of, 41
    physical sensations of, 41
frustration tolerance, 186–187
    documentation, 187
    low, characteristics of, 186–187
    low, risks associated with, 187
    problematic thought processes, 186

## G

gains, maintaining
    behavior markers (exercise), 244
    core beliefs, 244
    healthy lifestyle, 244
    new beliefs, 243
    tips, 245
gastrointestinal disorders, 231–232
    CBT stages for, 231–232
        core beliefs, 232
        education, 231
        problem solving, 232
        relaxation, 232
        stress management, 232
        thought processes, 232
    common symptoms, 231
    stress and, 231
Gate Control Theory, 224
generalized anxiety disorder, 168
goals
    anxiety disorder treatment, 168–169
    breaking down, 242
    fitness program, 81
    intentional, 101
    stress management, 145
goal setting, 55–62, 269
    coping flash cards (exercise), 61
    cost-benefit analysis (exercise), 60–61
    criteria, 55
    at first sessions, 270
    ladder rungs (exercise), 57–58
    maintaining progress, 61
        commitment levels, 61
        documentation, 61
    making sure goal is yours, 60
    motivation, defining of, 58
        lifestyle compromise, 58
        strategy, 58
        top rung of ladder, 58
    motivation, positive vs. negative, 59–60
        example, 59
        wording, 60
    pros and cons (cost-benefit analysis), 58–59
    SMART goal, 55–57
        attainable, 56
        coping statement, 57
        difficulty creating goal, 57
        example, 56
        measurable, 56
        questions, 56
        relevant, 56
        specific, 56
        timely, 56
        trouble reaching goals, 57

tips, 62
   behavior or feelings, 62
   broad goals, 62
   cost-benefit analysis, 62
   making the most difference, 62
   one behavior at a time, 62
graded therapy, facing fears with, 169
grief, 209–219
   ABC chart, use of, 214–215
      activating event, 214
      belief, 215
      consequence, 215
   beliefs challenged, 212–213
      crisis of identity, 213
      prayer, 213
      questions, 213
   benefit of CBT, 214
   change of priorities, 214
   customs, religious and cultural, 209
   definition of, 209–210
   effects of, 210
   feelings and behaviors, 210
   imaginal exposure, 216–217
      avoidance and, 216
      effectiveness of, 217
      example, 217
      story creation, 217
   length of, 219
   letter writing, 218
   losses, 213–214
      finances, 214
      relationships, 213
      responsibilities, 213
      routines, 213
   mixed emotions, 212
   new reality, 215
   permission to grieve, 211
   proactive steps, 214
      postponing decision-making, 214
      reaching out, 214
      talking to others, 214
   psychology of, 211–212
      emotions felt, 212
      guilt, 211
      mixed feelings, 212
   stages of, 209
   styles of grieving, 209
   thought process, 215–216
      dialogue, 215–216
      underlying belief, finding, 216
   uncomplicated vs. complicated, 218–219
   uniqueness of, 215
   waves of, 217–218
      first wave, 218
      management, 218
guided iCBT, 254, 256
guilt
   alternate words for, 42
   definition of, 42
   physical sensations of, 42

# H

*Happiness Now*, 110
Harrison, Vicki, 217
healthy emotions
   disgust, 42
   embarrassment, 42
   envy, 43
   frustration, 41
   irritation, 41
   nervousness, 40
   sadness, 41
   stress, 43
heart disease, 226–227
   causes of, 226
   CBT goals for, 226
   CBT techniques, 226–227
      activities, 227
      problem solving, 227
      stress management, 226
      thought restructuring, 227
   depression and, 226
   healthy lifestyle and, 226
high-risk situations, 249
hobbies, 79
Holden, Robert, 110
homework assignments, 269

hot buttons (anger), 183–185
    combating, 183
    coping statements, 184
    examples, 184–185

# I

iCBT. *See* internet-delivered CBT
ignoring the positive, 23, 35, 47, 57
illness, physical. *See* physical illness
image rescripting, 66–67
imagery. *See* visualization and imagery
imaginal exposure, 216
    avoidance and, 216
    effectiveness of, 217
    example, 217
    story creation, 217
inner narration, 91–98
    affirmations, 96
        believable, 97
        big picture, 97–98
        lying to yourself, 96–97
        tips, 98
    assessment (exercise), 95–96
    checklist, 95
        external statements, 95
        flexibility, 95
        focus, 95
        thoughts, 95
    negative narrations, 93
        perfectionist, 94–95
        self-critique, 94
        victim/blamer, 94
        worry, 93
    self-talk, 91–92
        automatic thoughts, 92
        belief in, 91
        form, 92
        negative, 91
        neutral, 92
        positive, 92
        ways, 91

    self-talk (exercise), 92–93
        cynical, 93
        example, 92
insomnia, 229–231
    behavioral changes, 229
        relaxation, 230
        sleep hygiene, 230
        sleep restriction, 229
        stimulus control, 230
        thought restructuring, 230
    chart, 230
    negative thoughts, 230
intentional goals, 101
International OCD Foundation (IOCDF), 257
internet-delivered CBT (iCBT), 253–262
    apps, 260–262
        Calm, 261
        CBT Thought Diary, 261
        Sanvello, 261
        What's Up?, 261
        Youper, 261
    benefits, 253, 255
        adherence, 255
        confidentiality, 255
        convenience, 255
        costs, 255
        time focused, 255
    disadvantages, 256
        difficulty asking questions, 256
        lack of therapist relationship, 256
    e-therapy websites, 258–259
        BetterHelp, 258
        Faithful Counseling, 259
        MDLIVE, 258
        Pride Counseling, 258
        Talkspace, 259
    locating programs, 256–258
        health insurance company, 257
        national organizations, 257
        potential programs, 257
        support group recommendations, 257
        website review, 257–258
    online programs, 259–260
        Beating the Blues, 260
        E-Couch, 260

Learn to Live, 260
Moodgym, 259
Online Therapy, 259
operation, 253–254
    conditions treated, 253
    guided iCBT, 254
    modules, 254
    primary forms, 253
    unguided iCBT, 254
pros and cons, 255
IOCDF. *See* International OCD Foundation
irritation
    alternate words for, 41
    definition of, 41
    physical sensations of, 41

## J

jealousy
    alternate words for, 43
    definition of, 43
    physical sensations of, 43
Jordan, Michael, 68
*Journal of Medicine and Life*, 222
*The Journal of the North American Menopause Society*, 228

## K

keynote behavior visualizations (exercise), 69–70
Kirtan Kriya meditation, 76
    mantra, 76
    meridian points, 76

## L

labeling, 25, 186
lapse
    definition of, 247
    reasons for, 249
    relapse vs., 247–248
        attitude, 248
        example, 247
learned emotions, 49–51
    conditioned emotional response, 51
    conditioning and, 49
    emotion chart, 50
    exposure techniques, 51
    fears, 50
    questions, 50
    similar situations, 51
letter writing, grief and, 218
losses
    finances, 214
    relationships, 213
    responsibilities, 213
    routines, 213
low frustration tolerance, 186
    characteristics, 186
    risks associated with, 187

## M

magical thinking, 173, 192–193
    disproving of obsessions, 193
    example (overcoming), 193
    postponing ritual completion (overcoming), 193
    practice (overcoming), 193
magnification, body image, 201
major depression, definition of, 42
mantra, 74
meditation, 74–76
    description, 74
    difficulty, 74
    mantra, 74
    purpose, 75
Meetup groups, 80
Melzack, Ronald, 224
memory, reframing of, 115
menopause, 230
    CBT strategies, 228
        mindfulness, 228
        relaxation and stress relief, 228
        thought restructuring, 228

coping statements, 228
medical interventions, 228
meta-emotions, 46
mindfulness, 83–90. *See also* present moment
   brain functioning during, 83
   breathing (exercise), 84
   definition of, 83–84
   diary (exercise), 90
   in everyday life, 89–90
      brushing teeth, 89
      eating, 90
      showering, 90
      waiting in line, 89
   meditation, exercise as, 151
   practice (exercise), 86
   presence in the moment, 86–87
      example, 87
      helpfulness of, 86
      practice, 87
      questions, 86
      refocusing exercise, 87
   presence in the moment, tips, 87–88
      conversations, 88
      deliberate movements, 87
      elimination of distractions, 87
      taking time to practice, 87
   role in CBT, 85
      distancing, 85
      space given, 85
      unproductive thought processes, 85
   rumination, 83
   thoughts, 84–85
      attitude, 84
      example, 84
      exercise, 88
      unfocused, 88
   thoughts, upsetting, 88–89
      acceptance, 89
      documentation, 89
      facts, 89
      questions, 88
   urges, controlling, 85–86
mind reading, 20–21, 47, 137, 174
   body image, 201
   perfectionism, 120

mixed emotions, 45, 51
   example, 45
   grief and, 212
   thoughts, 45
   unhealthy reactions, 45
motivation
   defining of, 58
      lifestyle compromise, 58
      strategy, 58
      top rung of ladder, 58
   finding, 241
      patterns, 241
      pros and cons, 241
   lack of, 158–159
      daily activity schedule, 158–159
      goal, 158
   positive vs. negative, 59–60
      example, 59
      wording, 60
muscle relaxation, 76–78
   description, 76
   exercise, 77–78
   feeling the difference, 77
MUSTerbation, 129
myths, 5–7
   childhood experiences, 6
   conditions helped by CBT, 6
   effectiveness, 6
   emotions, 6
   positive thinking, 6
   structure, 6
   underlying issues, 6

# N

National Association of Mental Illness (NAMI), 257
National Institute of Health, 229
negative automatic thoughts, 28–29
   examples, 28
   self-fulfilling, 29
negative motivation, 60
negative self-talk, 29–30

ABC chart, 30
    example, 29
    incomplete information, 29
negative thinking, 19
nervousness
    alternate words for, 41
    anxiety vs., 40–41
    definition of, 40
    physical sensations of, 41
new beliefs, development of core beliefs, 243
new beliefs, testing of, 99–106
    behaviors, 101–102, 105
        example, 101–102
        expectations, 105
        feedback, 103, 105
        observation, 104–105
        report card, 102–103
        reward, 105
        surveys, formal, 103–104
        surveys, informal, 104
    predictions, testing of, 106
    reality testing, 99–101
        example, 100–101
        experiment creation, 99–100
        experiment results, 100
        goals, 101
        review of original beliefs, 101

## O

observation, testing of behaviors through, 104–105
    example, 105
    proof of original theory, 105
obsessive-compulsive disorder (OCD), 189–197
    behavioral experiments, 193–194
        example, 193–194
        prediction decision, 194
        repeating of, 194
    building on successes, 196
        consistency, 196
        practice, 196
        setbacks, 196
    exposure therapy, 194–195
        anxiety level, 195
        imagery, 195
        list of actions, 194
        ranking of situations, 195
        urge to perform rituals, 195
    magical thinking, overcoming, 192–193
        disproving of obsessions, 193
        example, 193
        postponing ritual completion, 193
        practice, 193
    response prevention, 193
        definition, 193
        process, 193
    thought exposure (exercise), 192
        documentation, 192
        triggering of new obsessions, 192
    thoughts, 192
    tips for reducing rituals, 195–196
        flexibility, 195
        internal measurement, letting go of, 196
        stress management, 195
        thoughts, 196
        uncertainty, living with, 196
    triggers, identification of (exercise), 191–192
        during pandemic, 191
        example, 191
        ladder technique, 192
        log, 191
    understanding, 189–191
        common rituals, 190
        common themes, 190
        definition, 189
        example, 189
        powerlessness, 191
        seeking reassurance, 191
obstacles to progress, 235–242
    CBT tips, 242
        belief, 242
        breaking goals down, 242
        change of wording, 242
        jumping in, 242
        log, 242
        tracking of exercises, 242

common-sense strategies, 242
monitoring your progress, 241
more problems and feeling overwhelmed, 235–236
    battle, 235
    effectiveness of CBT, 235
    lifestyle change, 236
motivation, finding your (exercise), 241
    patterns, 241
    pros and cons, 241
reasons CBT doesn't work, 236
    analyzing everything you think, 238
    assumption about CBT, 237–238
    blaming others, 238–239
    expecting instant cure, 239
    failure to practice, 236
    fear of being uncomfortable, 240
    fear of failure, 240
    getting in your way, 239
    self-acceptance, meaning of, 237
    shame, guilt, and pride, 239–240
    trying to eliminate emotions, 237
OCD. *See* obsessive-compulsive disorder
*On Death and Dying*, 209
online CBT. *See* internet-delivered CBT
online CBT programs, 259–260
    Beating the Blues, 260
    E-Couch, 260
    Learn to Live, 260
    Moodgym, 259
    Online Therapy, 259
overgeneralization, 22, 47, 57, 104
    body image, 201
    self-esteem and, 111

# P

panic
    alternate words for, 41
    definition of, 40
    physical sensations of, 41
panic disorder, 168
passive-aggressive behaviors, 138

perfectionism, 117–125
    assessment (exercise), 118–119
    checklist, 121–122
    cost-benefit analysis, 123–124
    defining, 117–118
        areas, 117
        costs, 118
        effects on health, 118
        example, 117
    flexibility, 120
    overcoming (exercise), 125
    procrastination and, 124
        example, 124
        questions, 124
        strategies, 124
    rigid rules, revising, 121
        examples, 121
        physical environment, 121
    shades of grey, 122–123
        exercise, 123
        important standards, 123
        questions, 122
    thought patterns, 119
        absolutes, thinking in, 120
        black-and-white thinking, 119
        catastrophizing, 119
        mind reading, 120
        personalization and blame, 120
perfectionist, 94–95
    examples, 95
    problematic thought processes, 95
personalization, 22–23, 47
    body image, 201
    perfectionism, 120
phobias, 168
physical illness, 221–232
    chronic pain, 224–226
        adjunct therapy, 226
        brain interpretations, 225
        CBT treatment of, 225
        chart, 224
        coping factors, 224
        Gate Control Theory, 224
        statistics, 224
        therapies, 224

diabetes, 222–223
  CBT premise, 223
  clinical trial, 222
  complications, 222
  example, 223
  exercise, 223–224
gastrointestinal disorders, 231–232
  CBT stages for, 231–232
  common symptoms, 231
  decatastrophizing (exercise), 232
  stress and, 231
heart disease, 226–227
  causes of, 226
  CBT goals for, 226
  CBT techniques, 226–227
  depression and, 226
  healthy lifestyle and, 226
  how CBT helps, 221–222
  empowering treatment, 222
  goals, 221
  increasing treatment interaction, 222
  patient empowerment, 221
  psychological skills, development of, 221
insomnia, 229–231
  behavioral changes, 229
  chart, 230
  negative thoughts, 230
  relaxation, 230
  sleep hygiene, 230
  sleep restriction, 229
  stimulus control, 230
  thought restructuring, 230
menopause, 228
  CBT strategies, 228
  coping statements, 228
  medical interventions, 228
  mindfulness (exercise), 229
  procrastination (exercise), 229
physical sensations, as warning signs, 250
positive motivation, 60
positive thinking, myth about, 6
post-traumatic stress disorder (PTSD), 168
praise, 139
present moment. *See* mindfulness
problematic thought processes, 20, 137

anger, 177–188
  acceptance of fallibility, 185–186
  alternate words for, 41
  anger log (exercise), 178–179
  causes, 179–181
  complaints and requests (exercise), 181
  definition of, 41
  description, 177
  frustration tolerance, 186–188
  healthy vs. unhealthy, 181–182
  hot buttons, 183–185
  labeling (exercise), 186
  measurement of (exercise), 183
  physical sensations of, 41
  reframing of emotion, 185
  understanding, 177
black-and-white thinking, 21–22, 47, 174
  body image, 201
  perfectionism, 119
blame, 22–23, 179
body image, 201
  black-and-white thinking, 201
  fortune-telling, 201
  ignoring the positive, 201
  magnification, 201
  mind reading, 201
  overgeneralizing, 201
  personalization and blame, 201
catastrophizing, 20, 137
emotional reasoning, 24
fortune-telling, 21, 35, 137
frustration tolerance, 186
in goal setting, 57
identification of, 174
ignoring the positive, 23, 35, 47, 57
labeling, 25
mind reading, 20–21, 47, 137, 174
  body image, 201
  perfectionism, 120
overgeneralization, 22, 47, 57, 104
  body image, 201
  self-esteem and, 111
perfectionism, 95, 117–125
  absolutes, thinking in, 120
  assessment (exercise), 118–119

black-and-white thinking, 119
catastrophizing, 119
checklist, 121–122
cost-benefit analysis, 123–124
defining, 117–118
flexibility, 120
mind reading, 120
overcoming (exercise), 125
personalization and blame, 120
procrastination and, 124
rigid rules, revising, 121
shades of grey, 122–123
thought patterns, 119
personalization, 22–23, 47
body image, 201
perfectionism, 120
self-esteem, low, 94
self-talk adjustment and, 113
"should" statements, 137
stress, everyday, 147
thinking in absolutes, 24
victim/blamer, 94
worry, 93
procrastination, perfectionism and, 124
example, 124
questions, 124
strategies, 124
progressive muscle relaxation, 76–78
description, 76
exercise, 77–78
feeling the difference, 77
psychoanalysis, CBT compared with, 11
psychodynamic therapy, 264–265
CBT compared with, 11
characteristics, 265
criticism of, 265
premise, 264
psychotherapy, focus of, 7

## Q–R

rage
alternate words for, 41
definition of, 41
physical sensations of, 41
reactionary depression, 41
reality testing, 7, 99–101
example, 100–101
experiment creation, 99–100
experiment results, 100
goals, 101
review of original beliefs, 101
relapse, lapse vs., 247–248
attitude, 248
example, 247
relapse prevention plan, 250–251
coping statements, 251
exercises, review of, 250
skills, review of, 250
strategies, 251
supports, 251
thought logs, 251
relationships, improving, 127–134
blame, 127–128
abuse, 128
responsibility, 128
self-esteem, 128
thoughts, 127
communication skills, 131
listening, 132
nonverbal communication, 133–134
speaking, 132–133
cycle of unmet expectations, 131
compliments, 131
example, 131
demands, 129–130
ABC chart, 130
absolutes, thinking in, 129
examples, 129
expectations, 129
MUSTerbation, 129
questions, 130
statement disputes, 130

reaction, 128–129
    CBT suggestion, 128
    pattern, 129
    practical, 128
    ways, 128
sharing preferences (exercise), 130–131
relaxation techniques and strategies, 71–82
    activity journal (exercise), 81
    breathing, 71–72
        collapsed breathing, 72
        exercise, 72
        importance of, 72
        incorrect, 71
        proper, 71
        reverse breathing, 71
        shallow breathing, 72
    breathing (exercise)
        balloon breathing, 73–74
        deep breathing, 73
        feeling the difference, 73
        muscle development, 73
        sighing, 74
    finding time, 78
    fitness program, 81–82
        action plan, 82
        goals, 81
        research results, 81
        structured time, 81
    hobbies, 79
    meditation, 74–76
        description, 74
        difficulty, 74
        exercise, 75–76
        mantra, 74
        purpose, 75
    muscle relaxation, 76–78
        description, 76
        exercise, 77–78
        feeling the difference, 77
    physical activity and exercise programs, 81
    social activities, 80
        alternative gym, 80
        classes, 80
        community events, 80
        groups, 80
        places of worship, 80
        social media sites, 80
        volunteer work, 80
response prevention (OCD), 193
    definition, 193
    process, 193
reverse breathing, 71
Ross, Elisabeth Kubler, 209
ruminations, depression and, 160–161
    activities to stop process, 161
    conscious decision, 161
    documentation, 161
    "go-to" activity, 161
    thoughts surrounding, 160–161
ruminations, mindfulness and, 83

# S

sadness
    alternate words for, 42
    definition of, 41
    depression vs., 41–42, 155–156
    physical sensations of, 42
self-acceptance, 109–110
    components, 110
    difficulty of, 115
    happiness, 110
    levels of, 110
    meaning of, 237
    myth, 110–111
    obstacles to, 110
    responsibility, 110, 115
self-disclosure, 140
self-esteem, 109–115
    basing self-worth on one aspect, 111
    description of, 109
    external factors, measurement of worth on, 111
    low, 94
        examples, 94
        problematic thought processes, 94
    outdated self-image, 111
    overgeneralizing, 111
    self-acceptance, 109–110

components, 110
happiness, 110
levels of, 110
meaning of, 237
myth, 110–111
obstacles to, 110
responsibility, 110
self-assessment (exercise), 112
   statements, 112
   words, negative and positive, 112
steps to improving, 112–115
   accepting bad behavior, 114–115
   activities, 114
   comparisons, 113
   expectations, review of, 113
   mini action plan (exercise), 114
   self-talk monitoring and adjustment, 112–113
use of blame to protect, 128
self-talk, 28, 91
   automatic thoughts, 92
   belief in, 91
   exercise, 28
   form, 92
   monitoring and adjustment, 112–113, 115
      language, 113
      revised statements, 113
   negative, 29–30, 91
      ABC chart, 30
      example, 29
      incomplete information, 29
   neutral, 92
   positive, 92
   ways, 91
setbacks. *See* backsliding
shallow breathing, 72
shame
   alternate words for, 42
   definition of, 42
   physical sensations of, 42
shock
   alternate words, 43
   definition of, 43
   physical sensations of, 43
"should" statements, 137

sighing, 74
sleep
   breathing during, 72
   disturbances, depression and, 164–165
   restriction. *See* insomnia
SMART goal, 55–57
   attainable, 56
   coping statement, 57
   difficulty creating goal, 57
   example, 56
   measurable, 56
   questions, 56
   relevant, 56
   specific, 56
   timely, 56
   trouble reaching goals, 57
social activities, 80
   alternative gym, 80
   classes, 80
   community events, 80
   groups, 80
   places of worship, 80
   social media sites, 80
   volunteer work, 80
social anxiety disorder, 168
spontaneous imagery, 65
   example, 65
   forms of emotions and thoughts, 65
stereotypes, resisting, 34
stress
   alternate words, 43
   definition of, 43
   physical sensations of, 43
stress, everyday, 145–151
   definition of stress, 145
   exercise, 151
      beginning, 151
      endorphins, 151
      as form of mindfulness meditation, 151
      recommendations, 151
   problem solving (exercise), 148
   problems vs. problematic thinking, 147
      example, 147
      problematic thought processes, 147
      restructure of thinking, 147

stress management, goal of, 145
stressors, identification of, 146
    common stressors, 146
    documentation, 146
    examples, 146
stress reduction strategies, 149–150
    action steps, 149
    control and coping, 149
    example, 149
    getting help, 150
    muscle relaxation exercise, 150
    negative thought patterns, 150
    oasis, 149
    prioritizing, 149
    probability determination, 149
    relaxation techniques, 150
    stress-coping phrase, 150
    tech-free break, 150
    time for yourself, 150
unavoidable, 145
worksheet (exercise), 150–151
surveys
    formal, 103–104
    informal, 104
systematic desensitization, 169

## T

talk therapy, 264
telehealth specialist, 267
themes, 9
    anger/frustration, 9
    anxiety/nervousness, 9
    excitement/happiness, 9
    sadness/disappointment, 9
    shame/embarrassment, 9
theory behind CBT, 7–8
    empowerment, 7
    focus, 7
    premise, 7
    reality testing, 7
    steps, 8

therapist, working with, 263–271
    characteristics of good therapist, 268–269
        collaboration, 268
        concerns discussed, 268
        focus, 269
        goals, 269
        monitoring of progress, 269
        questions asked, 269
        referrals suggested, 268
        skills taught, 269
    cognitive behavioral therapy (CBT), 265–266
        benefits of, 266
        characteristics, 265
        criticism of, 266
        goal of, 266
    decision to seek help, 263–264
        guideline, 264
        reasons, 263–264
    finding a therapist, 266
    first session discussions, 268
    homework assignments, 269
    participation, 269
    psychodynamic therapy, 264–265
        characteristics, 265
        criticism of, 265
        premise, 264
    questions, 266–267
        background check, 267
        essential information, 266–267
        online forums, 267
        preference, 267
        reviews, 267
        telehealth specialist, 267
        website information, 266
    statistics, 263
    typical therapy session, 270–271
        discussion of issues, 270
        feedback, 271
        goal setting, 270
        practice, 270
        problem solving, 270
        questionnaire, 270
        reviews, 270
        skills introduced, 270

thinker types, 5
  outcomes, 5
  perspectives, 5
thinking. *See also* problematic thought processes
  in absolutes, 24
    perfectionism, 120
    relationships and, 129
  black-and-white, 21–22, 47, 174
    body image, 201
    perfectionism, 119
  magical, 173, 192–193
    disproving of obsessions, 193
    example (overcoming), 193
    postponing ritual completion (overcoming), 193
    practice (overcoming), 193
  negative, 19
  positive, 6
thought logs, 249, 251
thoughts, automatic. *See* automatic thoughts, assumptions, and core beliefs
thoughts and feelings, interpretation of, 15–26. *See also* problematic thought processes
  ABC worksheet, 25
  awareness of biased thinking, 25–26
  new beliefs, 18
  problematic thought processes, 20–25
    black-and-white thinking, 21–22
    blame, 22–23
    catastrophizing, 20
    emotional reasoning, 24
    fortune-telling, 21
    ignoring the positive, 23
    labeling, 25
    mind reading, 20–21
    overgeneralizing, 22
    personalization, 22–23
    thinking in absolutes, 24
  separating thoughts from emotions, 18–19
    avoidance, 19
    blame, 18
    creating new thought, 18
    decision-making, 19
    example, 18
    negative thinking, 19
    working backward, 18
  thoughts, feelings, and behaviors, 15–17
    ABC chart, 16
    emotions, 16
    example, 15
    initial thoughts, 16
    underlying thoughts, 16
  warning signs, 249
triggers, warning signs and, 249–250
  behaviors, 249
  emotions, 249
  high-risk situations, 250
  lapse, reasons for, 249
  monitoring of thinking patterns, 250
  physical sensations, 250
  thoughts, 249

# U

uncertainty, accepting, 172
  backward CBT approach, 172
  control, 172
  low tolerance for ambiguity, 172
  practice, 172
uncomplicated grief, complicated grief vs., 218–219
underlying issues, myth about, 6
understanding CBT, 3–13
  ABC chart, 8–9
    creation, 8
    purpose of, 8
    tip, 9
  automatic thoughts, 3
  benefits, 10
    adaptability, 10
    length of therapy, 10
    lesson learned, 10
    measurement of progress, 10
    structure, 10
    targeted skills, 10
  choosing CBT, 12–13
    CBT Readiness Quiz, 13
    checklist, 12

comparison with other forms of therapy, 11
   acceptance and commitment therapy, 11
   psychoanalysis, 11
   psychodynamic therapy, 11
core beliefs, 4–5
   perspectives, 5
   scenarios, 4
definition of CBT, 3
disadvantages, 10–11
myths, 5–7
   childhood experiences, 6
   conditions helped by CBT, 6
   effectiveness, 6
   emotions, 6
   positive thinking, 6
   structure, 6
   underlying issues, 6
themes, 9
   anger/frustration, 9
   anxiety/nervousness, 9
   excitement/happiness, 9
   sadness/disappointment, 9
   shame/embarrassment, 9
theory, 7–8
   empowerment, 7
   focus, 7
   premise, 7
   reality testing, 7
   steps, 8
thinker types, 5
   outcomes, 5
   perspectives, 5
unfairness, emotions based on sense of, 41
unguided iCBT, 254
unhealthy emotions
   anger, 41
   anxiety, 40
   contempt, 42
   feeling overwhelmed, 43
   guilt, 42
   jealousy, 43
   major depression, 42
   panic, 40
   rage, 41
   reactionary depression, 41

shame, 42
shock, 43
U.S. Centers for Disease Control and Prevention, 151, 156

## V

vasomotor symptoms (VMS), 228
victim/blamer, 94
   examples, 94
   problematic thought processes, 94
visualization and imagery, 63–70
   changing of focus, 67
   changing of image, 66–67
      image rescripting, 66–67
      memories, highly charged, 66
   coping skills, creation of, 68–69
      exaggerated visualizations, 69
      example, 69
      overwhelming situation, breakdown of, 69
      strategy, 68
   coping skills, creation of CBT techniques, 69
   emotional images, 64–65
      avoidance, 64
      desensitization, 64
      example, 64
      exercise, 64–65
      levels, 64–65
   imagery creation (exercise), 68
      athletes, 68
      practice, 68
   keynote-behavior visualizations (exercise), 69–70
   problem solving, 65–66
      change of image, 66
      example, 65
   spontaneous imagery, 65
      example, 65
      forms of emotions and thoughts, 65
   story completion, 67–68
      example, 67
      fleeting images, 68

testing of image, 66
    change of image, 66
    questions, 66
visualization, 63–64
    awkward situation, 64
    definition, 63
    details, 63–64
    example, 63
VMS. *See* vasomotor symptoms

# W–X–Y–Z

Wall, Patrick, 224
warning signs and triggers, 249–250
    behaviors, 249
    emotions, 249
    high-risk situations, 250
    lapse, reasons for, 249
    monitoring of thinking patterns, 250
    physical sensations, 250
    thoughts, 249
website review (iCBT), 257
websites, 258–259
    BetterHelp, 258
    Faithful Counseling, 259
    healthgrades.com, 267
    MDLIVE, 258
    Pride Counseling, 258
    Talkspace, 259
websites (CBT programs), 259
    Beating the Blues, 260
    E-Couch, 260
    Learn to Live, 260
    Moodgym, 259
    Online Therapy, 259
Woods, Tiger, 68
worry, 93
    example, 93
    excessive, cause of, 174
    problematic thinking processes, 93
    problem solving of, 171–172
    questions, 93
    script (exercise), 173
    theme, 93